Communication Skills for your

Nursing Degree

**CRITICAL
STUDY SKILLS**

Critical Study Skills for Nursing Students

Our new series of study skills texts for nursing and other health professional students has four key titles to help you succeed at your degree:

Studying for your Nursing Degree

Academic Writing and Referencing for your Nursing Degree

Critical Thinking Skills for your Nursing Degree

Communication Skills for your Nursing Degree

Register with **Critical Publishing** to:

- be the first to know about forthcoming nursing titles;
- find out more about our new series;
- sign up for our regular newsletter for special offers, discount codes and more.

Visit our website at: 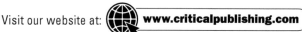 **www.criticalpublishing.com**

Our titles are also available in a range of electronic formats. To order please go to our website www.criticalpublishing.com or contact our distributor NBN International by telephoning 01752 202301 or emailing orders@nbninternational.com.

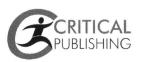

Communication
Skills for your
Nursing
Degree

CRITICAL
STUDY SKILLS

JANE BOTTOMLEY AND STEVEN PRYJMACHUK

First published in 2019 by Critical Publishing Ltd

British Library Cataloguing in Publication Data
A CIP record for this book is available from the British Library

ISBN: 978-1-912096-65-7

This book is also available in the following e-book formats:

MOBI: 978-1-912096-64-0
EPUB: 978-1-912096-63-3
Adobe e-book reader: 978-1-912096-62-6

Text and cover design by Out of House Limited
Project Management by Newgen Publishing UK
Printed and bound in Great Britain by 4edge, Essex

Critical Publishing
3 Connaught Road
St Albans
AL3 5RX

www.criticalpublishing.com

Paper from responsible sources

Contents

Acknowledgements

We would like to thank the many university and nursing students who have inspired us to write these books. Special thanks are due to Anita Gill and Patricia Cartney, and to Julia Morris at Critical Publishing for her support and editorial expertise.

Jane Bottomley and Steven Pryjmachuk

Meet the authors

Jane Bottomley

is a freelance writer, teacher and educational consultant. She is a Senior Fellow of the Higher Education Academy and a Senior Fellow of the BALEAP, the global forum for English for Academic Purposes practitioners. She has helped students from a wide range of disciplines to improve their academic skills and achieve their study goals, including 14 years as a Senior Language Tutor at the University of Manchester. Jane is the editor of the *Critical Study Skills* series, which covers nursing, education and social work.

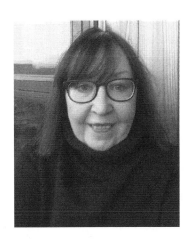

Steven Pryjmachuk

is Professor of Mental Health Nursing Education in the School of Health Science's Division of Nursing, Midwifery and Social Work at the University of Manchester and a Senior Fellow of the Higher Education Academy. His teaching, clinical and research work has centred largely on supporting and facilitating individuals – be they students, patients or colleagues – to develop, learn or care independently.

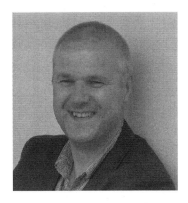

Introduction

Communication Skills for your Nursing Degree is the fourth book in the *Critical Study Skills for Nurses* series. The *Critical Study Skills for Nurses* series supports student nurses, midwives and health professionals as they embark on their undergraduate degree programme. It is aimed at all student nurses, including those who have come to university straight from A levels, and those who have travelled a different route, perhaps returning to education after working and/or raising a family. The books in the series will be of use both to students from the UK, and international students who are preparing to study in a new culture – and perhaps in a second language. The books also include guidance for students with specific learning requirements.

As well as technical/clinical skills, nurses and other healthcare professionals need to develop what are often described as 'soft skills', that is, communication skills and people skills. The terms 'oracy skills', 'interactional skills' and 'interpersonal skills' are also commonly used. Whichever terms are employed, the skills they describe are becoming increasingly important in university and professional settings. *Communication Skills* aims to support nursing students as they engage in vital oral and written communication activity in their nursing studies and professional lives. It focuses on improving general oral and written communication in professional life. It also provides guidance on public speaking, in particular, academic presentations, and covers the skills you need to participate in group discussions, especially seminars. It also provides guidance on communication with lecturers during tutorials, as well as discussing the skills required for successful networking in a range of contexts, including social media. If you require more information on academic writing, related to essays or dissertations, see another book in this series, *Academic Writing and Referencing for your Nursing Degree*.

Between them, the authors have many years' experience of both nursing practice and education, and academic study skills. All the information, text extracts and activities in the book have a clear nursing focus and are often directly linked to the **Nursing and Midwifery Council's Code**. There is also reference to relevant institutional bodies, books and journals throughout.

The many activities in the book include **tasks**, **reflections**, **top tips**, and **case studies**. There are also **advanced skills** sections, which highlight particular knowledge and skills that you will need towards the end of your degree programme – or perhaps if you go on to postgraduate study. The activities in the book often require you to work things out and discover things for yourself, a learning technique which is commonly used in universities. For many activities, there is no right or wrong answer – they might simply require you to reflect on your experience or situations you are likely to encounter at university or in your professional life; for tasks which require a particular response, there is an answer key at the back of the book.

These special features throughout the book are clearly signalled by icons to help you recognise them:

 Learning outcomes;

 Quick quiz or example exam questions / assessment tasks;

Reflection (a reflective task or activity);

 Case studies;

 Top tips;

 Checklist;

 Advanced skills information;

 Answer provided at the back of the book.

Students with limited experience of academic life and nursing practice in the UK will find it helpful to work through the book systematically; more experienced students may wish to 'dip in and out' of the book. Whichever approach you adopt, handy **cross references** signalled in the margins will help you quickly find the information that you need to focus on or revisit.

There are three **Appendices** (Academic levels at university; Key phrases in assignments; English language references) at the back of the book which you can consult as you work through the text.

We hope that this book will help you to become a successful communicator in all areas of your nursing studies and practice.

A note on terminology

In the context of this book, the term 'nursing' should be taken to include 'nursing, midwifery and the allied health professions', wherever this is not explicitly stated.

Chapter 1
Professional speaking skills

Learning outcomes

After reading this chapter you will:

- be aware of the particular characteristics of professional, as opposed to social, communication;

- develop your understanding of the role of oral communication in the context of nursing;

- be aware of the importance of oral communication skills as a part of the therapeutic relationship;

- be aware of strategies which can help you communicate and interact with patients, colleagues and third parties in a clear, appropriate and effective manner.

This chapter provides guidance to help you improve your oral communication skills in nursing and healthcare contexts. It will present a number of strategies to help you communicate and interact with patients and other parties in a clear, appropriate and effective manner.

Communication

A human language is essentially 'a signalling system' (Barber, 2000, p 2). The signals used include sounds, written symbols such as alphabets, and signs such as those in road signals, semaphore and the sign languages used by the Deaf Community. **Communication** can be defined as the transmission or exchange of information and ideas using these signalling systems.

Communication skills are one of the core skills of nursing, and they are central to the Nursing and Midwifery Council's Code (NMC, 2015). In this chapter, the focus is on general **oral communication**. Other chapters in this book deal with specific areas of oral communication which are important in academic life, ie presentations, seminars and tutorials. Chapter 6 focuses on the spoken and written communication skills required for successful networking. Chapter 2 looks at some areas of practical **written communication** in nursing. Another book in this series, *Academic Writing and Referencing for your Nursing Degree*, explores the writing skills you need to produce academic essays and dissertations.

The word 'communicate' presupposes the involvement of a person or persons on the receiving end of the transmission of information (eg the audience in a presentation) or participating in a two- or multi-way communication process (eg students participating in a seminar or nursing patients in clinical practice). For this reason, some people also use the word **interaction** when discussing

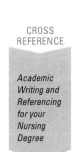

CROSS
REFERENCE

*Academic
Writing and
Referencing
for your
Nursing
Degree*

CROSS
REFERENCE

*Studying for
your Nursing
Degree,*
Chapter 3,
Becoming
a member
of your
academic
and
professional
community,
Graduate
attributes

these processes. **Communicative and interactional competence** is the focus of much current educational research (see for example Escobar Urmeneta and Walsh, 2017), and it is seen by many as key in the development of a range of **intellectual and interpersonal skills**. The development of these skills has become increasingly prioritised by universities in recent years. They form an important part of the '**graduate attributes**' promoted by universities, ie the **key transferable skills** which are believed to facilitate academic study while also preparing students for the world of work.

Professional communication

Professional communication is communication that occurs in a professional context rather than a social one. It is characterised by the fact that it is 'purposeful, ethical and has boundaries' (Jagger et al, 2015, p 47). It requires a high degree of self-awareness and a willingness to understand the lives and experiences of others. This means being aware of the gaps in your knowledge, the things you don't know or understand about the life of a person or people you are talking to. It also involves reflecting on your own values and beliefs. This includes trying to identify and acknowledge your own preconceptions and biases. We all grow up with social and cultural preconceptions and biases, some conscious, some unconscious. Being open to the realities of others and being more aware of your own preconceptions and biases can help you to communicate more sensitively and effectively.

Oral communication

As mentioned earlier, human communication is generally divided into spoken and written communication. Speech, however, is the 'primary form of language' (Barber, 2000, p 2). Speech is learned before writing, and while there are communities that have speech but no written form of their language, no human community has been discovered to have a written language without a spoken one (Barber, 2000). **Oral communication** obviously involves the voice, and the use of **verbal** elements such as sounds, words, phrases and sentences. But it involves much more than these. It comprises **non-verbal** elements such as facial expressions, body language and tone of voice. If you consider talking on the phone or writing an email, you can probably think of difficulties that can arise because of the absence of face-to-face contact with the person you are communicating with. For example, on the phone and in an email, you might need to be very careful when making a joke, as the person on the other end cannot see you smile (though it's perhaps sometimes possible to 'hear' a smile in your tone of voice on the phone). This is why we use 'emojis' ☺ ☹ ☺ in emails and text messages to friends to indicate emotions and pre-empt misunderstandings. However, when this tool is not available, in a more formal email for example, particular care is needed with regard to word choice and phrasing.

Michael Argyle, a renowned social psychologist, identified a number of **non-verbal cues** that humans use when interacting face to face (1988):

- facial expression;
- eye contact;

- posture;
- body space – proximity and closeness to others;
- gesture;
- touch;
- 'artefacts' – clothes and emblems and the way they make us look;
- paralanguage – *how* we say things rather than *what* we say, including intonation (the pitch and melody of the voice), vocal buffers ('oh', 'ah') and vocalisations (laughing, crying, groaning, muttering).

For nurses, it is especially important to be able to pick up on these cues in patients and other people. For example, not noticing or misreading such cues can result in a nurse failing to pick up on signs of escalating aggression, and this failure could even exacerbate such aggression. This is particularly important in areas of nursing where patients may be 'emotionally charged' such as accident and emergency, acute mental health wards and forensic care.

Communication in nursing

As a nurse, you will need to communicate with patients, as well as perhaps their carers, families and friends. You will also communicate with colleagues: some on a regular basis, others more intermittently. In addition, you will sometimes be required to interact with third parties such as social workers, translators and police officers.

As social beings, we perhaps instinctively feel that communication is an essential part of human relationships. It is generally accepted that interpersonal skills are important and that good communication and interaction should be encouraged in all aspects of life. But your own experience probably tells you that communication can often be tricky, and that people can quite easily misunderstand each other. Look at the following **case studies** and discuss what may have gone wrong, and how, perhaps, miscommunication could possibly have been avoided. Some of the issues raised will be discussed in more detail in later sections of this chapter.

Case studies

A

Reeta is a nurse working on a busy acute medical ward. A patient who felt nauseous at lunchtime missed lunch an hour ago, but she feels hungry now that the nausea has worn off. She asks Reeta if she could have something light, perhaps some toast and a cup of tea. Reeta is flustered because she has a thousand things to do, so she says to the patient (somewhat abruptly): 'Just give me ten minutes and I'll sort it.' Because she is so busy, Reeta forgets about this and goes on her break. When she returns from her break, she remembers the patient's request and asks the healthcare assistant to provide the patient with some tea and toast. It's now an hour and a half since the patient asked for something to eat, and when the healthcare assistant attends the patient with the tea and toast, the patient becomes really upset, saying that Reeta doesn't care about her.

1) What are the communication and interpersonal issues here?
2) How can Reeta resolve this communication issue now?

B

Jo is 15 years old. She was born male but currently identifies as female. Jo has been admitted to a young person's mental health unit following a serious suicide attempt. At the staff meeting, the unit manager says Jo was admitted because of self-harm arising from confusion over her gender identity. When Jo's keyworker asks Jo about this, Jo says she is not confused over her gender identity; Jo states she is female and has asked to be referred to by the pronouns 'she' and 'her'. Jo's appearance is gender-ambiguous and she dresses in gender-neutral clothing (jeans, t-shirts, trainers). Because of her appearance, some staff automatically and unintentionally refer to Jo as 'he' and 'him' within Jo's earshot. While this upsets Jo a little, she says she is more upset by those who refer to her as 'she' and 'her' without really meaning it. She says to her keyworker: 'At least those who accidentally refer to me as "him" are more genuine than those who say "her" through gritted teeth.'

1) What could make Jo say this? What aspects of paralanguage and body language might she be picking up on?
2) What is most important to Jo regarding the way people talk to or about her?

C

While on a medication round, a registered nurse asks a student nurse accompanying her to dispense 15ml of lactulose (a laxative) for a patient; the student mishears and gives 50ml of lactulose to the patient. While lactulose isn't particularly toxic, there are circumstances when mishearing the dosage of a drug can lead to serious problems or even fatalities.

1) What should the nurses have done in this situation?
2) What checks and balances are normally in place in to avoid these sorts of medication errors?

D

Jenny was involved in facilitating an inter-professional group which consisted of social workers, support workers, nurses and occupational therapists. In the middle of the session, Jenny made reference to CP – in social work this is an abbreviation for 'Child Protection'. She did in fact check herself, asking: 'Do we all use the term CP?' Everyone promptly nodded and the session continued. A little later, a discussion around risk management processes became rather confusing and the social workers and support workers seemed to be adopting a very different approach from the nurses and occupational therapists. They stopped for a moment to explore why the discussion had become so confused and found that although all the professions use the term CP, in fact it means different things in different professions. For social workers and support workers, CP is an abbreviation for 'Child Protection', whereas in the health professions, CP is an abbreviation for 'Cerebral Palsy'. Miscommunication was the result!

1) How could the participants have avoided misunderstandings over terminology?
2) What factors should be considered when using acronyms like 'CP'?

Discussion of case studies

A

The patient probably picked up on body language suggesting Reeta is flustered, which could make the patient feel like she is a nuisance and getting in the way of more important duties. Reeta also made a promise to the patient that was never fulfilled; this can lead to a breakdown of trust, something which is essential in the nurse–patient relationship. There is also the issue of delegating the task to an HCA who then has to deal with the aftermath of the situation. The best thing now would probably be for Reeta to apologise and provide an honest explanation – saying she forgot because the ward was so busy. It would be unhelpful for her to be defensive or try to justify her perhaps understandable lapse.

B

Jo is probably picking up on behaviour which she interprets as negative or judgemental. This is clearly not about what people say, as the people in question are using the language that has been agreed. However, perhaps their tone of voice or facial expression seems to convey that they are not comfortable or happy using this language because they do not understand or accept Jo's identification as female. It is clear that Jo understands that it might be difficult for people to adapt to her situation, and she accepts that people make mistakes; what is important to her is that people are genuine, even if that means showing their doubts or confusion.

C

The student should have checked the patient's prescription record with the registered nurse to see that the prescription was valid. She should also have double-checked ('Can I just check? Did you say 15ml or 50ml of lactulose?'). The registered nurse should have checked the dose after the student had poured it and before it was administered.

The **'five rights'** is a well-known way of understanding the checks and balances required for medication management. The five rights are:

1) right medication;

2) right dose;

3) right route;

4) right time;

5) right patient.

Even though this was a relatively minor medication error, it must be reported formally according to the clinical area's medication error policy. While this might cause some anxiety both for the student nurse and the registered nurse, it is necessary as most medication error policies are designed to prevent further errors happening rather than to discipline staff. However, if there are significant patient safety issues (eg a history of medication errors connected with this particular registered nurse), then disciplinary action of some kind would be likely.

CROSS REFERENCE

Academic Writing for your Nursing Degree, Chapter 5, Preparing your work for submission, Editing and proofreading your final text, Systematic treatment of names and titles

D

When we are part of a particular community, including academic and professional communities, it is often easy to assume that people outside that community know what we are talking about! Professionals sometimes use technical terms without providing an explanation, and this is particularly true of acronyms. We use acronyms because they are useful shorthand, but they are generally not accessible to people outside our immediate community. Jenny was right to check herself, but it would also have been useful to provide the full term at the outset of the discussion (as is the convention in academic writing).

Communicating with patients

Communication is one of the **'6Cs'** of nursing. In England, the 6Cs is a framework encompassing the values and standards that nurses are expected to work towards to ensure that patients receive high-quality care (NHS England, 2016). They comprise:

- care;
- compassion;
- courage;
- communication;
- commitment;
- competence.

Communication is, some would argue, perhaps the most important of these (see Barber, 2016) as, without good communication, it is difficult for nurses to adhere to the other values and standards in the list. Compassion, for example, requires communication that is perhaps more subtle: eye contact, tone of voice, proximity, etc. Rooting out poor care requires the courage to challenge established systems and staff who are often senior, and challenging these systems and staff requires robust communication skills. And nurses who lack communication skills are certainly not competent nurses: as Barber (2016) notes: 'Care may be compromised if nurses do not communicate well.' The following **reflection** touches on some important issues which will be discussed in the rest of this section.

Reflection

1) In what ways do you think communication most affects the patient experience?

2) What factors should be considered when talking to a patient? (Think about physical, environmental, cultural factors, for example.)

3) What do you need to consider when giving patients information about their condition or treatment?

4) How might you check that a patient has understood what they have been told?

5) What do you consider to be the values that should inform communication between a nurse and a patient?

6) Can you think of an incident from your own experience which could have been improved with better communication?

(adapted from Barber, 2016)

The therapeutic relationship

Nursing is a complex activity that simultaneously requires practical skills, intellectual skills and interpersonal skills. Communication forms an important part of the latter and, together with appropriate values, it is an essential part of a nurse's **therapeutic relationship** with a patient. Good communication between a nurse and a patient is dependent on the establishment of a relationship built on **trust** and **respect** and it is underpinned by personal attributes and values such as **empathy** and **compassion**. It can also be impacted by environmental factors such as décor, lighting and noise (Pryjmachuk, 2011). According to the Royal College of Nursing (nd), establishing good communication with patients helps patients feel:

- at ease;
- in control;
- valued.

Person-centred care

When considering how to communicate with patients, it is important to consider that nursing is today seen as part of an approach to medicine and healthcare which is known as **person-centred care**. This approach has wide support across the UK and in many other countries. It contrasts with disease or task-based care, which were more prominent in the past, and can still be observed today. Person-centred care is central to developing a therapeutic relationship which is founded on **trust**, **respect**, **rapport** and **collaboration**, and which aims to include patients in the assessment and planning of their care (Jagger et al, 2015). It is geared towards meeting their physical and psychological needs, and ensuring that they feel listened to. Its goal is to empower the patient and shift the locus of power or control so that it is more evenly distributed between patient and professional (Jagger et al, 2015), as opposed to the general ethos embraced historically, where the medical professional was 'in charge' and directing the interaction with the patient.

Being a good communicator

When speaking to patients (and to other parties) it is essential that you consider the **purpose** of your communication, ie what you want to achieve. It is important that your communication is **clear**, **meaningful** and **appropriate**, and that the patient, carer, etc is able to process and understand what you say.

The excellent #hellomynameis campaign, led by the late Kate Granger, outlines how simple it can be to improve communication.

It advises that you should:

- Always introduce yourself. In addition, it can be helpful to explain what your role is, eg:

  'Hello, my name is Charlotte [include surname if you wish]. I am a second-year student in children's nursing and I will be helping to look after you and your family while you're with us.'

- Ask patients (especially older patients) how they want to be addressed, eg:

  'Is it OK if I call you Mary?' or 'Do you prefer Mr Khan or Saeed?'

- Check that patients understand what you are saying to them, giving them ample opportunity to ask any questions.

You should also try to avoid:

- medical or technical jargon;
- acronyms and abbreviations that you might use as shorthand with medical colleagues;
- slang;
- terms which might cause offence or convey overfamiliarity.

There are a number of approaches and strategies which can help you to manage the way you communicate with patients, or at least help you to be more aware of the factors which can impact on that communication. Some of these are discussed below.

Rogers' core conditions

A well-known approach to patient care based on counselling principles (Rogers, 1980) establishes **three core conditions** as a prerequisite for successful communication as part of the therapeutic relationship:

- **Unconditional positive regard** – approaching people in a positive way and treating them with respect and warmth, irrespective of their presenting problems;
- **Empathic understanding** – putting yourself in the patient's shoes and understanding their perspective;
- **Genuineness** – being open and honest, and being yourself rather than presenting a professional or personal façade.

You may feel naturally inclined to such an approach. In fact, many people are drawn to professions like nursing because they believe in treating people in a way which presupposes these conditions. However, the establishment of these conditions also poses challenges. For example, nurses are sometimes faced with individuals who are known or believed to have behaved in a distasteful or criminal manner – individuals involved in gang violence or those who have perpetrated serious sexual offences for example. In these scenarios, it is important for a nurse to be able to reflect calmly on their role and responsibilities, and to focus on doing all they can to remain positive, empathetic and genuine. Another challenge is to distinguish empathy from sympathy. Feeling sorry for someone is not the same as trying to understand their perspective. Furthermore, looking or sounding sympathetic is not necessarily a true sign of genuine concern; it can sometimes mask indifference or even annoyance.

Reflection

Think of some of the clichés often used in nursing and ask yourself if they truly convey empathy – or even genuine sympathy, eg:

1) 'I'm sure everything will be alright.'

2) 'It must be awful for you.'

3) 'I'm sorry, you'll have to ask the doctor/nurse in charge.'

Can you think of some alternative ways of expressing sympathy and empathy that are perhaps more genuine?

Discussion of reflection

1) 'I'm sure everything will be alright.'

Will it? How do you know? Compare with:

> 'There have been lots of people who've had similar difficulties as yours and we've been able to help almost all of them.'

2) 'It must be awful for you.'

This can sound almost dismissive. Compare with:

> 'I've never had that sort of experience myself and can't imagine what you are going through but it's clear you must be going through a very difficult time. Is there any way I can help?'

3) 'I'm sorry, you'll have to ask the doctor/nurse in charge.'

This is a default 'I don't know what to say' statement for many.
Compare with:

> 'I'm sorry, I don't know but I can try and find out for you if you'd like.'

Egan's SOLER framework

As mentioned earlier in the chapter, non-verbal aspects of language such as those identified by Argyle (1988) are as important as the words we use. Another approach that has been very popular in nursing is Egan's **SOLER** framework (1975), which represents elements of non-verbal communication which are believed to facilitate and enhance the therapeutic relationship:

  S – **sit squarely** in relation to the person, ie face them

  O – adopt an **open** posture, eg don't cross arms or legs

  L – **lean** slightly towards the person

  E – maintain **eye contact** with the person

  R – **relax**

This framework could help create the right atmosphere and put people at ease during clinical interviews or when breaking bad news. However, it is not without its challenges. Being overly conscious of achieving the first four in the list could possibly have an adverse effect on the last one! That is to say, worrying too much about perfecting SOLER could make the interaction seem wooden or forced. Stickley (2011) has criticised SOLER, claiming that it misses out on the value of touch and the 'therapeutic space' in therapeutic interactions. Stickley proposes **SURETY** as an alternative:

S – **sit at an angle**

U – **uncross legs**

R – **relax**

E – maintain **eye contact**

T – appropriate use of **touch**

Y – use **your intuition**

Active listening

A well-known strategy believed to aid communication in contexts such as nursing is **active listening**. By definition, the term '*active* listening' challenges the idea that listening is a passive process in which one person (the speaker) 'does something' and the other person (the listener) simply 'absorbs' information. The process of 'active' listening involves paying close attention to the person speaking, noticing the words they use, their tone of voice, their facial expression and their body language, and reflecting on what all of this conveys about what they are thinking and how they are feeling. It requires you to be 'present' in the moment (Rogers, 1961), to listen carefully and show genuine interest, and to make every attempt to understand the patient's point of view.

Active listening may involve the following (adapted from Jagger et al, 2015).

- Verbal communication, for example:
  - acknowledging what the other person is saying, and signalling your own reflective state, often by using words such as 'yes', 'right', 'I see', or even recognisable sounds such 'ah' and 'uh um';
  - clarification techniques such as checking that you have interpreted the speaker's message correctly or directly questioning;
  - restating, paraphrasing or summarising the speaker's message to check understanding and provide a focus.
- Non-verbal communication, for example:
  - non-verbal aspects of 'paralanguage', such as intonation;
  - body language, such as posture, eye contact, facial expressions, gestures and touch. (See Argyle's 'non-verbal cues', 1988, presented earlier in the chapter.)
- Being quiet and perhaps still, creating space for the other person to think and express themselves.

Active listening is important in nursing for a number of reasons.

- It can help nurses in their assessment of patients.

- It is an effective way of conveying the empathy and genuineness necessary for the therapeutic relationship, as it conveys to an individual that they have the full attention of the person they are talking to.
- It can support people who find it difficult to express themselves in what may seem to them to be a stressful situation.
- It can help nurses to manage a volatile or highly emotional situation.
- It can help nurses to know when and how to engage with the patient, and to respond in the right way, be it through eye contact, a knowing look, a smile or, in the right circumstances, a touch.

Task

Identify the active listening techniques employed by the nurses in the following exchanges with patients.

1)

Patient: 'Some days I can walk and move about quite easily. Then other days my joints are very stiff and painful and I even find it difficult to get up and get dressed. I never know how I'm going to feel when I wake up.'

Nurse: 'Uh um, so your pain levels and mobility vary from day to day.'

2)

Patient: 'There are days when I just can't face getting up in the morning. No one can imagine what it feels like.'

Nurse: 'So, when you have these days, can you try to explain to me more what it feels like?'

3)

Patient: 'I was diagnosed with diabetes five years ago and had to start taking medication.'

Nurse: 'Was it type 2 diabetes? That's the sort of diabetes that develops over time? Have you brought your medication with you?'

Patient: 'Yes, that's right; I've my tablets here… they are called 'met' something.'

Nurse: 'Metformin?'

Patient: 'That's it!'

Nurse: 'So let me just make sure I've got this right. You were diagnosed with type 2 diabetes five years ago, and you've been on metformin ever since.'

4)

Nurse: 'Can you tell me a bit more about your diet at the moment?'

Patient: 'Well it's not good, especially when I'm down. I eat too many biscuits and cakes, and too much chocolate. I wish I could eat more healthily but it's so hard.'

Nurse: 'What do you consider to be a healthy diet? We could have a look at what you eat over a typical week and see how you can increase healthier foods and decrease the less healthy ones.'

Questioning techniques

It is impossible to carry out a nursing assessment without asking questions. Most of these questions will be routine, but it's likely you will at some point have to ask patients and those around them difficult questions. Depending on the situation, you may have to ask questions related to issues such as money, sexual behaviour, substance abuse, personal relationships or domestic and sexual violence. Where the safeguarding of a child or vulnerable adult is an issue, you will have no choice but to ask these sorts of questions.

In general terms, it is worth being aware of the different types of question you might ask – both with difficult questions and the more routine ones – and to consider how appropriate or effective each type may be in a given situation.

The three main types of question in English are discussed below.

Closed questions

These are questions such as:

'Did you take your medication this morning?'
'Have you spoken to the doctor?'

They anticipate an answer of 'yes' or 'no', and are therefore sometimes referred to as 'yes/no-questions'. They are particularly useful when you need information quickly, for example in an emergency situation. They can also be used to 'add structure' to a conversation (Jagger et al, 2015, p 44). However, in the wrong situation, they may be seen to be 'leading', ie influencing the patient's answer in a way that is ultimately unhelpful (Jagger et al, 2015, p 44). And closed questions are not always the best way of asking difficult questions: asking 'Have you been sexually abused?' is very different from asking 'So you wear dentures?'

Open questions

These are questions such as:

'What pills and how many of them did you take this morning?'
'Where do you feel the pain?'

They usually begin with a 'question-word' such as 'what/where/when/who/why/how', and are therefore sometimes known as 'wh-questions'. They do not presuppose a particular answer, and they can elicit both long and short answers, eg:

'Where do you feel pain?'	'Here.'
	'In my lower back.'
	'It depends. Sometimes my lower back hurts. Other times, I feel pain in my hips and thighs. Sometimes it shoots down my leg.'

Open questions can also be used to follow up on closed questions to elicit additional information. They are also particularly good for initiating conversations about difficult topics:

'If you're OK with it, could you tell me how you came to be evicted?'

Searching/Probing questions

These are open questions that are intended to elicit a deeper understanding of a situation (Jagger et al, 2015). They are less specific than the open questions above and provide space for a patient to open up and help direct the conversation, for example:

'How are you feeling today?'
'What kind of upbringing did you have?'

Probing questions are good as follow-on questions for difficult topics:

'OK so you were evicted because you ran up debts on your rent and ignored the letters from your landlord asking you to get in touch? How have you handled money and paying your rent and other bills in the past?'

Reflection

Think about how you might phrase questions when you need to find out about a person's:

- substance abuse;

- financial difficulties;

- sexual behaviour;

- living conditions;

- criminal behaviour.

(Pryjmachuk, 2011, p 65)

Therapeutic touch

Touch is often used in complementary therapies such as massage and reflexology, but it also plays a more general role in nursing communication. This could be touching or holding the hand of a patient, or perhaps hugging a relative who has been bereaved. It can be effective, and it may cut through the use of words in many situations. However, it is important that individual preferences and cultural considerations are taken into account. Certain individuals may be uncomfortable with physical contact for any number of reasons, perhaps relating to mental illness or experience of abuse, or merely out of personal preference. And in some cultures, certain types of touching – or any touching at all – may be taboo. The key is to be alert to the feelings and reactions of the patient and to respond with understanding.

Being human!

The frameworks, strategies and techniques outlined above can be very helpful. Even if you don't adopt them systematically and completely, familiarity with them can still help make you more aware of the issues involved when you are communicating with patients. As you might expect, emerging as they do from fundamental nursing principles, they share much common ground. They prioritise certain values and attributes such as respect, empathy, compassion, genuineness and patient-centred care. However, as already discussed, it can sometimes be challenging to follow the requirements of these frameworks in certain situations. It can also be difficult to hold multiple considerations in your head at the same time while remaining natural, present and 'human' in your interaction. If you do feel a bit awkward or overwhelmed, it is perhaps a good idea to start with trying to focus on some simple communicational principles as outlined in the following **top tips** box.

Top tips

Keeping it simple

- **Pay attention** to the person you are speaking to and **listen** to what they say. This should go a long way towards helping you achieve the outcomes desired by Egan, Rogers and proponents of active listening. Paying attention and listening should, for example, help make your physical stance open and engaging without you thinking about it too much. It should also mean that you pick up on the perspective and feelings of a patient.

- When you speak and ask/answer questions, the important thing is to **make yourself understood** to the patient, using simple words and short sentences where possible. Give the patient the time and the opportunity to process information and make sure you **check** that they have done so. This includes taking account of those whose first language is not English, or who may have a disability which affects communication. It is also a consideration if English is not your own first language: don't worry about minor grammar mistakes or the fact that you have an accent (everyone has an accent – a French accent, a South African accent, an American accent, a southern English accent, a Mancunian accent, etc); focus on being clear. Note these sections of the NMC Code (2015):

  - 7.1 Use terms that people in your care, colleagues and the public can understand.

- 7.2 Take reasonable steps to meet people's language and communication needs, providing, wherever possible, assistance to those who need help to communicate their own or other people's needs.
- 7.3 Use a range of verbal and non-verbal communication methods, and consider cultural sensitivities, to better understand and respond to people's personal health needs.
- 7.4 Check people's understanding from time to time to keep misunderstanding and mistakes to a minimum.
- 7.5 Be able to communicate clearly and effectively in English.

- **Put compassion at the heart of your communication and interaction with a patient.** Compassion can be defined as 'a sensitivity to suffering in self and others, with a commitment to try to alleviate and prevent it' (Gilbert, nd). In other words, it means *noticing* (a central feature of active listening) distress in those you are caring for, and doing what you can to prevent or reduce it. If you approach all communication and interaction with compassion, with a commitment to noticing and alleviating distress, you will go a long way towards meeting the necessary conditions of the therapeutic relationship.

Here are some other **top tips** to help you in particular nursing contexts.

Top tips

Completing assessment forms

If using a standard nursing assessment form, try to make the assessment more like a **natural conversation** rather than a questionnaire. This will help you build up **rapport** with the patient. It might be important that all of the questions on the assessment are asked but they need not be in the order listed or necessarily asked exactly as written. Make use of additional reflecting ('So, let me just check…') and probing statements ('Tell me a bit more about that…') to ensure that the assessment is accurate.

Top tips

Delivering bad news

It is always difficult to deliver bad news. It requires the personal attributes of courage, kindness and compassion. It is important to be clear on what is or isn't possible, and to be careful not to give false hope (Jagger et al, 2015). It is also important to listen carefully to people's questions and concerns, perhaps employing some of the active listening techniques discussed earlier in the chapter. This includes being ready to respond appropriately to the reaction of the person you are delivering bad news to, offering a kind word or, if appropriate, using touch.

Developing good communication skills through practice and feedback

If you are reading this book, it is hopefully because you believe it can help you to improve your communication skills. This book aims to raise your awareness of the issues involved and strategies that you may find helpful. However, this book, or any other book, is only part of the story. As with any skill, the best way to improve is through **practice** (Figure 1.1). This is the case whether you are learning an academic or professional skill, or whether you are learning a new language or how to dance the tango. And for practice to be truly effective, it needs to be accompanied by **feedback** (Figure 1.1), ie advice on how you can improve in the future.

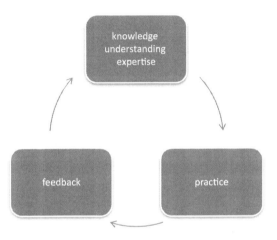

Figure 1.1: The learning cycle

As a student nurse, you will receive feedback from lecturers, mentors, peers and patients. In order to benefit from feedback, you should be aware of how to interpret it and use it. You should approach feedback in a positive manner, with the intention to reflect on it seriously and carefully – there is always room for improvement, no matter how experienced a person is. Focus on both strengths and weaknesses, and try to identify small steps that you can take to improve in one or two specific areas – you can't put everything right at once. As a student nurse, you will be supervised in many aspects of your training. However, if you realise that you feel uncomfortable or lacking in confidence in a particular area of practice, you should actively seek supervision so that you can obtain the feedback you need in order to improve.

CROSS REFERENCE

Studying for your Nursing Degree, Chapter 6, Assessment, Feedback on academic work

Role-play

One way of practising your communication skills on your degree programme is through **role-play**. People have different reactions to role-play, but it is an established part of many nursing degree programmes, so you need to be able to participate in it effectively. It is therefore worthwhile reflecting on how you feel about role-play and how you can best approach it if you find it difficult.

Reflection

1) What experience have you had of role-play?

2) Which of the following would you associate with your experience of role-play? Why?

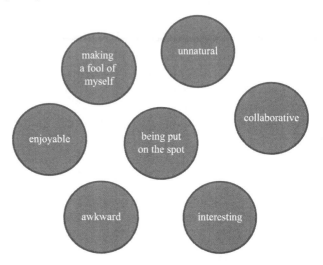

3) If you chose some or mostly negative associations, consider how you might adopt a more positive approach. You could start by recognising that role-play is designed to test out situations in a safe environment; it is better to make mistakes in role-play and learn from them than it is to be overconfident with real patients.

Communicating with others

As noted earlier in the chapter, as a nurse, you will have to communicate with a range of people in addition to patients. You will be required to talk to patients' carers, family or friends, both informally and in more formal contexts. You will also communicate with colleagues and third parties such as other members of the healthcare team, social workers, housing officers, translators or police officers. This requires the same communication skills which you need to communicate effectively with patients (thus, these skills are *transferable skills*). Sometimes the roles may be reversed, in that you may need to answer questions from others rather than ask them.

Summary

This chapter has explored the role of oral communication in nursing, including both verbal and non-verbal features. It has examined the role of oral communication in the therapeutic relationship and presented some approaches, strategies and techniques which could help you to communicate more clearly, appropriately and effectively with patients and other parties.

References

Argyle, M (1988) *Bodily Communication*. 2nd ed. London: Methuen.

Barber, C (2000) *The English Language*. Canto edition. Cambridge: Cambridge University Press.

Barber, C (2016) Communication and the 6Cs: The Patient Experience. *Nursing Times*, 30 May [online]. Available at: www.nursingtimes.net/roles/adult-nurses/communication-and-the-6cs-the-patient-experience/7005176.article (accessed 23 October 2018).

Egan, G (1975) *The Skilled Helper: A Systematic Approach to Effective Helping*. Belmont, CA: Thompson Brooks/Cole.

Escobar Urmeneta, C and Walsh, S (2017) Classroom Interactional Competence in Content and Language Integrated Learning. In Llinares, A and Morton, T (eds) *Applied Linguistic Perspectives on CLIL* (pp 189–206). Amsterdam: John Benjamins.

Gilbert, T (nd) Compassion in Education: Embedding and Assessing Compassion in the University Curriculum [online]. Available at: https://compassioninhe.wordpress.com (accessed 23 October 2018).

Hellomynameis [online]. Available at: www.hellomynameis.org.uk (accessed 19 September 2018).

Jagger, C, Iles-Smith, H and Jones, J (2015) Nursing Therapeutics. In Burns, D (ed) *Foundations of Adult Nursing* (pp 35–62). London: Sage.

NHS England (2016) *Leading Change, Adding Value: A Framework for Nursing, Midwifery and Care Staff* [online]. Available at: www.england.nhs.uk/leadingchange/about (accessed 19 September 2018).

NMC (Nursing and Midwifery Council) (2015) *The Code: Professional Standards of Practice and Behaviour for Nurses and Midwives* [online]. Available at: www.nmc.org.uk/globalassets/sitedocuments/standards/nmc-standards-for-competence-for-registered-nurses.pdf (accessed 23 October 2018).

Pryjmachuk, S (2011) The Capable Mental Health Nurse. In Pryjmachuk, S (ed) *Mental Health Nursing: An Evidence-Based Introduction* (pp 42–72). London: Sage.

Rogers, C (1961) *On Becoming a Person: A Therapist's View of Psychotherapy.* Wiltshire: Redwood Books.

Rogers, C (1980) *A Way of Being.* New York: Houghton Mifflin.

Royal College of Nursing (nd) Why Communication is Important [online]. Available at: https://rcni.com/hosted-content/rcn/first-steps/why-communication-important (accessed 23 October 2018).

Stickley, T (2011) From SOLER to SURETY for Effective Non-Verbal Communication. *Nurse Education in Practice*, 11(6): 395–98 [online]. Available at: www.sciencedirect.com/science/article/pii/S1471595311000618 (accessed 19 September 2018).

Chapter 2
Professional writing skills

Learning outcomes

After reading this chapter you will:

- have developed an understanding of a range of professional writing contexts in nursing;

- be aware of how to follow the guidelines on record keeping contained in the NMC Code;

- be better able to write clear, well-organised reports;

- be better able to write official correspondence;

- be aware of how to produce effective information leaflets.

This chapter will help you to understand the kind of writing that is expected of you as a professional nurse. It will help you to achieve different writing goals and to develop your professional writing skills.

Writing basics

When writing any text, the key considerations are **audience** and **purpose**.

- Who will be reading the text?
- What is your purpose in writing the text?

With respect to academic essay writing, the concepts of audience and purpose are explored in detail in another book in this series, *Academic Writing and Referencing for your Nursing Degree*. Audience and purpose should also guide the writing that you need to do as part of your nursing practice. This includes record keeping, writing reports, developing patient information leaflets and writing official correspondence such as letters and emails to patients, statutory/ non-statutory agencies or other health professionals. Each of these will be discussed in more detail below.

CROSS REFERENCE

Academic Writing and Referencing for your Nursing Degree, Chapter 1, Academic writing: text, process and criticality, Approaching a writing assignment

Record keeping

As discussed in Chapter 1, effective communication skills are essential in nursing and effective communication cannot be achieved without good record keeping. Good record keeping plays a vital role in promoting patient safety and continuity of care

(Royal College of Nursing, 2015) and Section 10 of the NMC Code (2015: 9) outlines the importance of creating and maintaining clear and accurate records:

10 Keep clear and accurate records relevant to your practice.

This includes but is not limited to patient records. It includes all records that are relevant to your scope of practice. To achieve this, you must:

10.1 Complete all records at the time or as soon as possible after an event, recording if the notes are written some time after the event.

10.2 Identify any risks or problems that have arisen and the steps taken to deal with them, so that colleagues who use the records have all the information they need.

10.3 Complete all records accurately and without any falsification, taking immediate and appropriate action if you become aware that someone has not kept to these requirements.

10.4 Attribute any entries you make in any paper or electronic records to yourself, making sure they are clearly written, dated and timed, and do not include unnecessary abbreviations, jargon or speculation.

10.5 Take all steps to make sure that all records are kept securely, and

10.6 Collect, treat and store all data and research findings appropriately.

Look at the following case studies and decide which parts of Section 10 of the Code are most relevant in each case.

Case studies

A

Shelagh, the ward manager, undertook an annual personal development review (PDR) with one of her junior staff nurses, Kinga. In this meeting, Shelagh and Kinga discussed what had gone well in the time since the last PDR, what hadn't gone so well, and what developmental needs Kinga might need in the future. Shelagh kept some handwritten notes of the PDR meeting but didn't get round to writing it up until two weeks later. When Shelagh sent the written report to Kinga for review, Kinga sent it back saying it needed amending as there were some inaccuracies in it.

B

Scott, a second-year student nurse on placement in a nursing home, wrote some brief notes about a patient he was looking after in the patient's paper records. He got his supervisor to countersign the notes but then realised he had written the notes in the wrong patient's records. He took the notes out of the file, destroyed them securely and rewrote them in the correct patient's records.

C

Acacia Ward uses an electronic record-keeping system for its patients' notes. The Trust that runs Acacia Ward has a shortage of IT staff and it takes weeks for staff to get a login and password for the system. Amy, a new staff nurse, has just started work on the ward but doesn't have a password yet. Reza, one of the other staff nurses, lets Amy use his login and password.

D

Debra is a newly qualified mental health nurse working in an inpatient mental health ward. She has been identified as the named nurse for a new patient, Anthony, who was brought to the ward by the police. The police tell Debra it's been a struggle getting him there as he was very resistant and aggressive. Debra carries out the admission interview with Anthony and writes up the notes immediately afterwards. In it, she writes 'aggressive and resistant to admission'. A week later, Anthony seems more settled and asks to see his notes. He questions why he's been described as aggressive and resistant, stating that he told her at admission that he was unhappy that he had been forcibly brought into hospital against his will, especially since he was worried about his dog being left alone. He feels the statement gives people a false impression of him.

Discussion of case studies

A

Shelagh left it too long (10.1) between the PDR meeting and the write up and this led to some inaccuracies (10.3) that Kinga had to point out. It would have been better if Shelagh had written up her records of the meeting soon after it had taken place.

B

Scott's supervisor should have checked that the notes were for the right patient before countersigning to ensure they were not countersigned while they were technically inaccurate (10.3). Scott may have had good intentions in removing the notes and securely destroying them, but if the notes were a continuation of previous notes for the other patient, he may have destroyed important existing records. To ensure compliance with 10.2, Scott should have deleted his entry by drawing a line through the notes he had made and writing something underneath it like 'written in error'. This should then be signed (with date and time) by Scott and countersigned by his supervisor.

C

This will contravene 10.4, as the system will record any notes that Amy makes in Reza's name. It could also technically be considered as falsification (10.3). Until Amy gets a login of her own, she should not be making any notes in the electronic system. If there continues to be unacceptable delays with obtaining her own login, she should escalate the issue with her line managers (or senior managers in the Trust if this fails) because both she and Reza are risking their NMC registrations with this behaviour.

D

While Debra has complied with 10.1, having written the notes up immediately after the admission interview, she may have breached 10.3 in relation to accuracy because she wrote simply 'aggressive and resistant to admission'. A more accurate entry might be: 'the police officers who brought Anthony in stated that he was aggressive and resistant to admission'. In addition, some context might be useful, eg 'Anthony remained relatively calm throughout the admission interview and explained he was very upset and had "put up a fight" because he did not want to go to hospital and was worried about who would look after his dog'.

If 'aggressive and resistant to admission' was what was actually recorded in the notes, Debra would now need to write something extra to ensure that Anthony's subsequent concerns were recorded, eg 'Anthony approached me to ask why he's been described as "aggressive and resistant" in his notes. I explained that this was how the police had described him. He feels the statement gives people a false impression of him as he is not normally aggressive and felt it was an appropriate response to "put up a fight" when he was being taken to hospital against his will and was worried about the welfare of his dog.'

The Academy of Royal Medical Colleges (2018) has produced some guidance for writing outpatient clinic letters to patients but the principles in this guidance are useful for general medical and nursing records.

- Use English rather than Latin terms, eg 'paracetamol as required' rather than 'paracetamol prn'.
- Avoid medical phrases like 'the presenting complaint was...' Instead, write 'the patient attended the clinic/ward/service because...'.
- Explain acronyms or, better still, write the term in full, eg electro-convulsive therapy rather than ECT, chronic obstructive pulmonary disease rather than COPD.
- Pay particular attention where the recipient of information is a child or young person or if the recipient has a visual impairment.
- Avoid stigmatising phrases: 'is living with diabetes' is better than 'is a diabetic' and 'has been diagnosed with schizophrenia' is better than 'is schizophrenic'.

Some of these guidelines are discussed in more detail later in the chapter.

Use and misuse of abbreviations and acronyms

Section 10.4 of the Code advises against the use of unnecessary abbreviations. However, there are some abbreviations and acronyms which are common knowledge and which can therefore be used in records. It is a case of balancing speed (abbreviations and acronyms save time) with accuracy and transparency.

Note:

An **acronym** is the short form of a multi-word term, often a proper name. Acronyms are usually formed by using the first letter of each word, but they are sometimes adapted slightly to make them more readable or memorable. Examples include:

BBC (British Broadcasting Corporation)

NICE (National Institute for Health and Care Excellence)

An **abbreviation** is formed by simply shortening a word; this is usually indicated by a full stop. Examples include:

approx. (approximately)

etc. (from the Latin *et cetera*)

Task

1) What do the abbreviations and acronyms below stand for?

2) Which of them are acceptable and which are best avoided in record keeping? Give reasons.

eg	A&E	prn	CAMHS
TLC	NHS	Ca	RCN

Discussion of task

eg – acceptable

This means 'for example' and it is commonly used in both professional and everyday writing.

TLC – best avoided

This is generally used for 'tender loving care', a euphemism meaning a patient is dying; it should be avoided because not only does it mask the truth from patients and relatives, but there are also other medical terms it could be confused with, eg 'total lung capacity'.

A&E – acceptable

This is a well-known abbreviation for the Accident & Emergency department. A&E departments were formerly known as 'casualty' departments and their renaming was an attempt to prevent misuse by the public. Although using the abbreviated A&E is acceptable, it might be better to use its full name or the shorter 'emergency department' since this retains the spirit of the name change from 'casualty'.

NHS – acceptable

This is a very well-known abbreviation for the National Health Service. It rarely needs explanation within the UK but may need to be explained to international audiences.

prn – best avoided

This is from the Lain *pro re nata* and is used to mean 'as required' in relation to medication, eg 500mg paracetamol prn. Most doctors and nurses know what prn means but lay people may not. There is an argument that 'as required' should be used instead of prn.

Ca – best avoided

This is sometimes used as an abbreviation for carcinoma (cancer) but is also the chemical abbreviation for calcium; ambiguity here could create anxieties for patients or relatives. For example if a patient sees 'Ca+ in bloods' in their notes, it might actually refer to a blood test for calcium but could easily be misinterpreted as a blood cancer.

CAMHS – probably best avoided

This is a well-known acronym for Child & Adolescent Mental Health Services that is very common among mental health professionals and mental health service users. However, it is seen as an increasingly outdated and stigmatising acronym. Many people working in this area prefer instead to use 'Children and Young People's Mental Health Services', a term that doesn't really lend itself to acronym use.

RCN – acceptable

Almost everyone in nursing knows that this abbreviation stands for the Royal College of Nursing.

Avoiding jargon

Section 10.4 of the Code warns against the use of 'jargon'. When you habitually use certain technical terms, it can be hard to put yourself in the shoes of someone who does not have the same technical knowledge as you. This could apply to someone outside your professional community, or even a colleague who has not been working in the same area as you. It could also apply to patients.

As an example, the prefixes 'hyper' and 'hypo' are frequently used in medical terminology. To the public, they sound very similar but actually have completely opposite meanings, with 'hypo' meaning 'below' or 'low' and 'hyper' meaning 'above' or 'high'. Thus, 'hypotension' means 'low blood pressure' and 'hypertension' means 'high blood pressure'; likewise, 'hypoglycaemic' means 'low blood sugar' while 'hyperglycaemic' means 'high blood sugar'. Confusing hypo and hyper can have serious consequences as the following example from Frankel and Vecchio (2010) illustrates.

Case study

During a busy morning a patient in the intensive care unit was noted by a doctor to have high blood pressure requiring immediate intervention (severe hypertension). The doctor mentioned to the nurse that the patient was hypertensive and gave a spoken order for 5 mg of hydralazine [a vasodilator which relaxes the arteries]. Unfortunately the nurse misheard the doctor and thought he had said that the patient was hypotensive. As a result the drug was misinterpreted and 5 mg of metaraminol [a vasoconstrictor which 'tightens' blood vessels] was administered … The result was that the patient was given a drug with the opposite effect of the desired one, at a dose 10 times the usual and resulting in treatment worsening the problem it was intended to reduce.

Frankel and Vecchio argue that we should simply use plain English 'low' and 'high'. What do you think?

Task

Improve this entry in the nursing notes to take into account the guidance provided in the preceding sections.

Mrs Sutton was admitted to Ward 37 by sn Rosenbaum at 1 o'clock. Complaining of melana and haematemesis. Has h/o of GI problems. Current meds only otc 75mg Zantac prn. FBC. For GI scope asap.

Confidentiality

You are probably aware of new legislation on data protection. If you have been in employment or volunteering for a charity, you have probably been asked to complete training to bring you up to date with this legislation; and if you use the internet, you cannot fail to have noticed that the number of boxes you are required to tick has been on the up. This is because, on 25 May 2018, the EU General Data Protection Regulation (GDPR) came into force alongside a new UK Data Protection Act. This new legislation is concerned with 'person identifying information' (PII), such as a person's name and address, and the way this information is collected, stored and used. The legislation requires that organisations and individuals:

- collect and retain only the minimum amount of PII data necessary;
- are transparent with people about how they are using their data;
- provide people with choices with regard to this usage where possible;
- keep the data they collect secure;
- retain data only for as long as it is required.

As a student nurse, you will be required to follow data protection guidelines issued by your host university, the NHS and healthcare providers. In particular, you need to be aware that breaches of GDPR can have serious financial consequences (big fines) for the organisations involved. While many breaches are accidental, part of the reasoning behind GDPR was to try to force organisations (through big fines) to ensure their staff take the processing of PII more seriously. Few data protection breaches in healthcare are a result of criminality or downright negligence; most are in fact down to carelessness, eg:

- leaving confidential paperwork in unattended places like on a desk in an unlocked office;
- leaving an unencrypted electronic device with personal information on it in unattended places, eg losing your mobile with work email on a bus;
- emailing personal information to the wrong person, eg sending an email reply to all rather than a single recipient;
- sending a letter to the wrong address;
- posting pictures or information on social media without checking for personal information, eg photos from a ward Christmas party in which patients can be seen in the background.

Such lapses can have serious consequences. In order to avoid them, keep yourself up to date with the NMC Code and any organisational policies on data protection. In addition, remind yourself to slow down and be particularly careful whenever you are handling sensitive personal information.

Countersigning

In your clinical practice, a registered nurse may delegate record keeping to you so that you can have valuable practice in documenting care. The registered nurse is required to ensure that any student nurses under their supervision are competent to undertake this activity and that it is in the best interests of the patient for record keeping to be delegated (Royal College of Nursing, 2015). For this reason, the registered nurse who is supervising must provide a countersignature until the student nurse is 'deemed competent at keeping records', which is normally at the point of graduating and entering the NMC Register. The countersignature must be for activity they have witnessed and/or can validate.

A model for remembering the principles behind good record keeping

The Code provides guidelines based on key principles. The following keyword models may help you to keep these principles in mind:

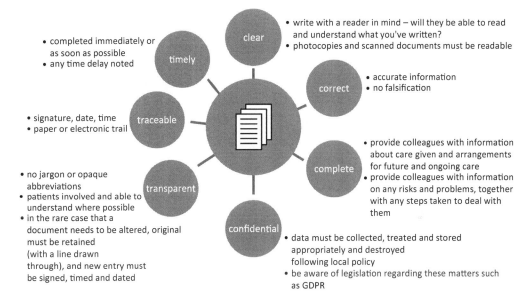

Figure 2.1: Principles of record keeping
(Some additional information taken from Royal College of Nursing, 2015)

Writing reports

A report requires you to present and analyse information, and sometimes to provide recommendations. In some ways, report writing is similar to essay writing in that it requires a high degree of planning based on a clear understanding of the following.

- Why are you writing the report? (purpose)
- Who will be reading it? (audience)

This second question can be slightly difficult in report writing. An academic essay usually has only one type of reader, ie a university lecturer. However, a report could potentially have one or several types of reader, eg professionals and the general public. When planning and writing a report, it is very important to bear in mind all the potential readers. Sometimes, two reports are written, one for a professional audience and one for the general public. This is very common in healthcare research. In addition, if a report is particularly long, a shorter version of the report, called an 'executive summary', tends to accompany the longer report. This allows busy professionals (or, indeed, the general public) to get the gist of the main aspects of the report without having to read all of it.

As well as good planning, a report requires a process of careful drafting and editing, just like an academic essay.

A report must have a clear objective and a very precise structure. When writing a report, first check if there is a standard template that you are expected to adopt. This might include details such as:

- specific headings;
- whether sections should be numbered;
- requirements for a glossary (a list of definitions of key terms).

If there is no template, format the report logically so that it is consistent and easy to navigate.

During their normal working lives, every qualified nurse will have to write a report of some sort. This could be:

- a report related to health and safety or specific clinical issues;
- a report related to the line management of staff;
- a report proposing an innovation or change in practice or even a reorganisation of a clinical service;
- a report for a case conference on a specific patient or service user.

Task

Familiarising yourself with some official reports from professional nursing bodies such as the RCN can help you to understand the typical format and style of official reports in nursing. Below are some extracts from an RCN report: 'International Workforce in the UK after Brexit: Nursing Issues' (2018).

 1) Read the extracts quickly (ignoring the gaps for now) just to get the main idea and decide which part of the report they come from by matching them to the report headings:

- Background
- What are the issues?
- What needs to happen?

A

Post-Brexit immigration arrangements will undoubtedly impact on nursing which is why the RNC is seeking to a) _____ them. The UK has a b) _____ nursing workforce with circa 15% of our registered nurses coming from overseas.[5]

B

The UK's domestic workforce supply has not a) _____ rising patient need, nor the increasing demand for care outside hospital settings. In the NHS in England alone there are b) _____ 40,000 vacancies.[1] Scotland has vacancy c) _____ of 4.5%[2] and there is an d) _____ vacancy rate in Northern Ireland of 6.9%.[3] In Wales, e) _____ national vacancy rates are not collected and published, the high spend on f) _____ _____ does demonstrate a need for additional nurses in Wales.

C

We believe that from an overall workforce perspective, the post-Brexit immigration system should:

- Support the education, recruitment and a) _____ of the nursing workforce as a whole, to b) _____ the UK has sufficient numbers of staff with the right skills and attitudes to deliver the c) _____ health and care services the population needs.

2) Now read more carefully and complete the extracts using the words and phrases listed below:

> kept pace with agency nurses shape retention approximately
> diverse vital rates estimated although ensure

3) Read the whole report (it's very short) here: www.rcn.org.uk/professionaldevelopment/publications/pub-007181. Do you find it easy to read? Why is this?

4) What do you notice about the way it is written and presented? Consider:

- how it is formatted – the page layout, headings, the use of bullet points, the use of bold and colour;

- the length and content of paragraphs;

- the style and language used.

Top tips

Report writing

1) Bear in mind the **purpose** of the report and keep the prospective **reader** at the forefront of your mind while writing. Ask yourself if they will be able to navigate the report easily, extract the main message, and understand any important details.

2) The purpose of the report and the needs of the reader should determine all **formatting** choices.

- Is the layout reader friendly? Does it allow the reader to navigate sections easily?

- Is the font and use of colour, bold, etc conducive to easy reading?

- Are the headings meaningful? Do they relate exactly to the content beneath them? Could they be shorter and simpler?

- Could bullet points help the reader to read a list more easily?

3) You want the reader to take the content seriously so presentation should be to professional standard.

4) Think about how figures and tables may help you to convey your message more clearly.

5) Sentences and paragraphs should be kept quite short wherever possible, and each paragraph should stick to one main idea, preferably indicated in the first sentence.

6) Language should be fairly formal and kept simple wherever possible. Check spelling, grammar and punctuation carefully; again, this is important if the report is to appear serious and professional to the reader.

7) Use colons and semi-colons to present lists, eg:

Respondents identified several areas of concern:

- funding;
- staffing;
- safety.

CROSS REFERENCE

Academic Writing and Referencing for your Nursing Degree: Chapter 4, Language in use, Grammar, spelling and punctuation

Task

Improve the report extract below by correcting mistakes in spelling, grammar and punctuation.

Key objective of any future imigration system should be ensure that UK can attract and retain the highly skill nursing workforce required to provide quality care, which meets patient need. International recruited nurses have made an important contribution to this goal; while enhancing the cultural diversity of the proffession and facilitate a rich exchange of skills and experience.

(adapted from Royal College of Nursing, 2018; mistakes added)

CROSS REFERENCE

Record keeping

Writing official letters

As mentioned earlier in this chapter, the Academy of Royal Medical Colleges (2018) has issued useful guidelines for writing to patients. These advocate a 'plain English' approach, avoiding Latin terms, medical jargon, and obscure or confusing acronyms and abbreviations. They also promote transparency and inclusivity, and avoidance of stigmatising language.

Nurses often have to write official letters or emails to other health or social care professionals (eg discharge summaries to GPs or referral letters to clinics or services) or to government agencies.

Task

Read the example letter from a community mental health nurse to a GP and answer the questions.

1) Which address is that of a) the sender and b) the recipient?

2) What does 're' (first line of the letter) mean?

3) The letter starts with 'Dear Dr Other' and ends with 'Yours sincerely'. When would you end a letter with 'Yours faithfully'?

4) What is the purpose of the letter?

5) Who will read the letter?

6) Is the language used in the letter suitable for all readers?

7) Does the letter follow the Academy of Royal Medical Colleges guidelines (2018) discussed earlier?

Anytown Community Mental
Health Team
Anytown Partnership NHS Trust
The Cedars
Short Lane
Anytown AT10 3AA

Dr A N Other
The Clinic
24 High Street
Anytown AT10 1AA
10 September 2018

Dear Dr Other

Re: Mr Andrew Person (date of birth 10/10/75), 7 Long Road, Anytown AT10 1BB

Following your referral to the community mental health team, I visited Mr Person on the afternoon of Thursday 7 September 2018.

At Mr Person's request, I interviewed him in the presence of his wife, Andrea. Mr and Mrs Person were both upfront about Mr Person's mental health and the impact it was having on their day-to-day lives.

You explained in your referral that you felt Mr Person had severe health anxiety that had consequently led to some degree of agoraphobia. In interviewing and assessing Mr Person, I would agree with you. Mr Person ruminates constantly about bodily symptoms and is convinced he is going to have a heart attack or stroke or that he has developed cancer. He told me it all seemed to have started when his father-in-law died suddenly six months ago from a heart attack. His ruminative thoughts are often worse in the early hours of the morning, which is having a detrimental effect not only on his sleep but on his wife's too. As part of our routine mental health assessment, we ask about suicidal ideation. Mr Person expressed no suicidal thoughts though both he and his wife stated that they were 'exhausted' by it all.

He told me that you had referred him for a variety of physical health tests recently, all of which have come back negative, but these have not reassured him, even though he knows that, rationally, they should. He is fully aware that the root of his problems is anxiety-related but he is unable to prevent negative, intrusive thoughts about his health and a general fear of death. He is afraid to go out in case he collapses and has been off work now for three months. Mrs Person says it is having a significant toll on her health as she is exhausted and feels guilty about leaving him at home when she goes out to work.

Mr Person told me he is not taking any prescribed, over the counter, or illicit medication though he smokes around 20 cigarettes a day. He drinks very little, perhaps a glass of wine or two a week with meals.

He has explored self-help options via the internet but he told me he often got distracted and ended up looking at information about other health conditions, which only made his anxieties worse. I feel he would benefit from the supported cognitive-behavioural programme that the community mental health service offers. He is open to this and we should be able to start the programme in the next week or two.

In case you are not aware, our programme usually lasts around eight weeks. We normally write to the referring practitioner again once the programme has completed. The team has a reasonable success rate with this programme, although some people do find it unsuitable; if this is the case, or if Mr Person's mental health deteriorates before the end of the programme, I will write to you sooner.

If you have any questions in the meantime, please contact me on 0161 333 2222 or by emailing cmht@anytown.nhs.

Yours sincerely
Christine Nurse
Senior Community Mental Health Nurse
cc. Mr A Person

Top tips

Using the right salutation and sign-off in official letters and emails

There are two ways to start an official letter, and two ways to end it. The conventions governing the choice of salutation and sign off can seem a little old-fashioned and rather arbitrary, but it is worth knowing about them. In short, if you know the name of the person you are writing to, start with 'Dear Mr _____' or 'Dear Ms/Miss/Mrs _____' and end with 'Yours sincerely'; if you do not know the name of the recipient, start with 'Dear Sir' or 'Dear Madam' and end with 'Yours faithfully'.

OPENING	CLOSING
Dear Mr Brown Dear Ms Gonzalez Dear Mrs Chowdry	Yours sincerely
Dear Sir Dear Madam Dear Sir or Madam	Yours faithfully

A good way to remember this is by noting that you don't use two 's's' ('sir' and 'sincerely') together. With regard to the use of Ms/Miss/Mrs, it is common practice today to use the generic form 'Ms'. However, if you are writing to someone who you know prefers 'Miss' or 'Mrs', then you should probably go with their preference.

Writing patient information leaflets

Nurses will sometimes be asked to produce information leaflets. These might, for example, provide information on a particular condition for patients. It might be used as written back-up for a conversation you've had with a patient.

As with all the writing discussed in this chapter, to write information leaflets, you need to have a clear idea of the **purpose** of the leaflet, and the needs and expectations of the target **reader** (as well as patients, the leaflet might be read by family members, carers, etc).

A good place to start is to make a list of all the questions which a patient, or those around them, might have about their condition (Turnbull, 2003). A study by Coulter et al (1998; reported in Turnbull, 2003) found that patients want to understand:

- the causes of the problem;
- the treatment options;
- things they can do themselves;
- risks and benefits.

Once you have listed your questions, you need find authoritative and reliable information to go about answering those questions – the NHS and NICE are good starting points. You then need to consider how you can make this information accessible to a patient with no expert knowledge.

It is important that information leaflets are not over-technical, too impersonal or too formal. The reader needs to feel comfortable reading the leaflet. It should not be intimidating to the reader, but neither should it talk down to them.

Top tips

Writing information leaflets

1) The tone should be conversational – imagine explaining something face to face. Use personal pronouns ('You might want to consider making changes to your diet') and avoid impersonal passive sentences ('Changes in diet are considered beneficial').

2) The language should be simple and readable. This might mean using short sentences where possible and explaining any difficult or technical words in plain English ('pre-eclampsia – a condition that can occur during pregnancy. It can cause high blood pressure and damage to organs.').

3) The writing should be concise – avoid any words or phrases which are unnecessary, so that the reader can extract the main message easily.

4) Choose your words carefully – your language should be 'reassuring and non-alarmist' (Coulter, 2003, cited in Turnbull, 2003, p 27). This might mean avoiding too many negative words. However, you should also be careful not to understate problems and risks.

Summary

This chapter has explored the different kinds of writing expected of you as a professional nurse. It has looked at how to write records, reports, correspondence and information leaflets, with a focus on achieving your aim, bearing the reader in mind, and writing in a clear, appropriate and effective manner.

References

Academy of Royal Medical Colleges (2018) Please, Write to Me: Writing Outpatient Clinic Letters to Patients. Guidance [online]. Available at: www.aomrc.org.uk/wp-content/uploads/2018/09/Please_write_to_me_Guidance_010918.pdf (accessed 23 September 2018).

Coulter, A, Entwistle, V and Gilbert, D (1998) *Informing Patients: An Assessment of the Quality of Patient Information Materials*. London: King's Fund.

Frankel, A and Vecchio, P (2010) Commonly Used, Easily Confused: Let's Eliminate Hyper and Hypo. *BMJ*, 341: c5867.

NMC (Nursing and Midwifery Council) (2015) *The Code: Professional Standards of Practice and Behaviour for Nurses and Midwives* [online]. Available at: www.nmc.org.uk/globalassets/sitedocuments/nmc-publications/nmc-code.pdf (accessed 19 August 2018).

Royal College of Nursing (2015) Record Keeping: The Facts [online]. Available at: www.rcn.org.uk/professional-development/publications/pub-006051 (accessed 12 August 2018).

Royal College of Nursing (2018) International Workforce in the UK after Brexit: Nursing Issues [online]. Available at: www.rcn.org.uk/professional-development/publications/pub-007181 (accessed 30 September 2018).

Turnbull, A (2003) How Nurses Can Develop Good Patient Information Leaflets. *Nursing Times*, 99(21): 26–7 [online]. Available at: www.nursingtimes.net/Journals/2012/11/09/v/f/g/030527How-nurses-can-develop-good-patient-information-leaflets.pdf (accessed 23 September 2018).

Chapter 3
Academic presentations and public speaking

Learning outcomes

After reading this chapter you will:

- be able to approach public speaking with greater confidence;

- be better able to select suitable content for academic presentations and organise it effectively;

- be better able to produce visual aids which support and enhance your academic presentations;

- have developed strategies to enable you to deliver effective academic presentations on the day;

- have an idea of the different types of presentation you might be asked to do at university (individual, group, poster).

Public speaking forms an important part of academic and professional life, and can also feature more widely in our personal lives.

Reflection

1) Have you done any of the following?
   - given an academic presentation;
   - spoken at a political meeting or community event;
   - given a commercial presentation;
   - spoken on TV or radio;
   - spoken on social media, eg in a podcast or a video;
   - done any of the above in a second language.
2) How did you feel about doing these things?
3) How did you prepare?

Oracy skills in academic study

The skill of **public speaking** is an example of what are sometimes referred to as 'oracy skills', ie skills that involve speaking and listening, as opposed to 'literacy skills', which involve reading and writing. There is growing interest in the role of oracy skills in education (see Mercer et al, 2017), and they will undoubtedly form an important part of your degree programme, as well as your future professional life.

For you, as an undergraduate nursing student, the oracy skills that you will develop and be assessed on at university will probably include giving academic **presentations**, both individually and in groups, and participating in group **seminars**. The nature and function of the oracy skills you employ in these different contexts will vary. In a presentation, you will be aiming to present ideas that you have worked through, crafted and refined. In contrast, in a group seminar, you may be trying to express ideas that you are still getting to grips with, testing them to see if they hold water, perhaps adapting them as you listen to what others have to say. So oracy skills are not only a way of demonstrating what you have learned; they are also a learning tool, a way of helping you to process knowledge and work through ideas. They are thus an essential part of critical thinking.

This chapter will help you to understand the principles behind public speaking, in particular, academic presentations, and it will provide strategies that you can adapt to your own circumstances and learning preferences. The next chapter will help you to participate more successfully in seminars.

The following **case studies** demonstrate how people's experience of public speaking and academic presentations differs. The issues they raise will be discussed subsequently in this chapter.

CROSS
REFERENCE

*Critical
Thinking
Skills for
your Nursing
Degree*

CROSS
REFERENCE

Chapter 4,
Participating
in group
seminars and
meetings

Case studies

Look at the student comments below. Do any of them reflect your own experiences and feelings about public speaking and presentations?

1) 'I quite enjoy speaking in front of an audience.'

2) 'I much prefer giving presentations to writing!'

3) 'I feel sick for a week before I give a presentation.'

4) 'I have butterflies for the first five minutes of a presentation, then I usually relax and enjoy it.'

5) 'English is not my first language so I find it really difficult to present in English and I worry about making mistakes with grammar and pronunciation.'

6) 'I dread questions from the audience – they always throw me.'

7) 'The lecturers on the course ask us to use PowerPoint but I worry that I don't know how to use it as well as other students on my course.'

Giving effective academic presentations

Students arrive at university with varying degrees of experience of academic presentations.

Reflection

1) What experience do you have of:
   - giving academic presentations in front of fellow students, teachers or lecturers?
   - presenting academic papers at conferences?
   - listening to academic presentations?
2) In your opinion, what makes:
   - a good presentation?
   - a bad presentation?

There is no one answer to the question of what makes a good presentation, but the following section provides:

- strategies, advice and tips which can help you prepare an academic presentation and deliver it effectively on the day;
- opportunities for reflection so that you can work out what might work best for you;
- tasks to help you start putting some of what you learn into practice.

Presenting style

There is no single style which defines a good presentation. For example, some people are very animated and entertaining while others are quieter and rather business-like. Both styles, as well as other ways of presenting, can be effective.

Reflection

1) Think back to any time you have been in the audience at a talk, speech or presentation. What kind of presenting styles did you notice? Which did you find most effective?
2) How would you describe your own style of presenting? Has it changed at all with any experience you've gained?

Whatever your personal style, the audience, and your assessors, are generally looking for a presentation which is:

- professional and well prepared;
- clear and easy to follow;
- engaging and interesting.

To ensure that your presentation has these qualities, you need to do a lot of work beforehand. When you see a presentation go smoothly, it is easy to forget the intense effort that has usually gone into making this happen – just as an elegant swan might appear to be gliding effortlessly across the water while their feet are working furiously beneath the surface!

The following sections will elaborate on the things that you can do to prepare your presentation and make sure things go as smoothly as possible on the day. There is also advice on how to cope when things don't go quite as smoothly as you'd hoped (it can happen to us all!).

Audience and purpose

When writing, the most important considerations are *your purpose in writing* and *the person reading your text*; likewise, when presenting, the most important considerations are *your purpose in presenting* and *the people listening to you*.

CROSS REFERENCE

Academic Writing and Referencing for your Nursing Degree, Chapter 1, Academic writing: text, process and criticality

Reflection

1) Discuss the last presentation you gave. What was the purpose of the presentation? Who were the audience?

2) Do you think you achieved what you set out to do?

3) How do you think the audience responded to you?

4) Is there anything you would do differently next time? Why?

If you have ever been in an audience where you felt lost or bored, it could well have been because the presenter misjudged the context of their presentation, and was perhaps thinking more about what *they* wanted to say rather than what *you* wanted or needed to hear. Try to avoid making that same mistake in your own presentations by thinking very carefully about the context of your presentation and preparing it with your **purpose** and a particular **audience** in mind. In your case, you are likely to be presenting to your lecturers and fellow students. This might be in the form of a 'formal' presentation, where you stand at the front of the room and present to an audience seated in front of you, often as part of your assessment. Or it might be a presentation to a group of your peers in a seminar situation, which could also be assessed. Your purpose in the former situation is primarily to demonstrate your knowledge and understanding of the topic. In the latter situation, your purpose could be to set up and lead a group discussion. As you advance in your studies, you may be presenting your research, either to lecturers and fellow students at university, or more widely at conferences. In all cases, the most important thing is to adapt to the context, whatever it is, and to cater for the needs and expectations of the people who will be sitting in front of you.

CROSS REFERENCE

Chapter 4, Participating in group seminars and meetings

Research and preparation

Preparation, involving research and the selection, organisation and presentation of information and ideas, is essential to a good presentation.

Reflection

1) What factors do you consider when selecting content for a presentation?

2) What do you aim to achieve when organising your content? What do you think are the principles of good organisation?

3) Do you ever go over time when giving presentations? If so, why do you think this is?

CROSS
REFERENCE

Appendix 1,
Academic
levels at
university

It is important that you research the topic carefully and, particularly at levels 5 and 6, *critically*. Your lecturers will be looking for you to show that you are in full command of the material. This doesn't necessarily mean knowing every last detail about every aspect of the topic. In fact, your lecturers will expect you to be selective and to acknowledge any areas of doubt. This is part of being a *critical* student.

Selecting and processing information and ideas

When researching a topic, you are likely to encounter a great deal of information. It is therefore important that you establish the **scope** of your presentation, based on purpose and audience, **select** material which is appropriate, relevant and, hopefully, interesting for your audience, and then **process** that material so that your audience will be able to digest it easily. When selecting which material you will choose to cover and how much detail you will go into, it is important to consider the following questions.

- How much is your audience likely to know about the topic? It's important that you **pitch your presentation at the right level**. You don't want to talk down to people in the room, but neither do you want what you say to go completely over people's heads. Consider which concepts and terminology you can assume knowledge of, and which you may need to define and explain. Remember, if the concept or terminology was new to *you*, then it's likely that you will need to explain it to other students at the same level. And even though your lecturers are very likely to already know about the concepts and terminology in your presentation, they will be expecting you to explain a great deal in order to demonstrate your own knowledge and understanding. And remember, even lecturers don't know everything! They often learn something new from student presentations and are very happy to do so.

- How can you **make the topic accessible** to your audience? Some aspects of the topics you present may well be complex and difficult to understand. Think about how you can help the audience to process information, perhaps by breaking things down or explaining things in a step-by-step fashion. You may also be able to support your explanations with diagrams, or use vivid examples to clarify a point.

- How can you **make the topic interesting** for your audience? Have you ever listened to a presentation where the presenter seemed intent on telling you every last detail of a topic without regard for what you, the audience, might want or need to know? This is often a sign that presenters have not considered the audience at the planning stage. They could be very competent presenters, but if they have only thought about *what they want to say*, rather than *what this particular audience might want or need to hear*, they will find it hard to engage the audience. Effective presenters, on the other hand, think about what is appropriate and relevant for the people in front of them and then think about how they can convey these things in the most accessible, interesting way possible.

- How can you **say what you have to say in the time available**? Practise giving your presentation several times, and time yourself to make sure that the content you have selected fits the time you have been allotted. Be careful when adding or deleting content as this can affect the coherence of your presentation. One easy way to extend or shorten a presentation can be to add or delete discrete examples, as these can be easy to slot in or take out without affecting the general flow of information and ideas. Remember, it is unprofessional to go over time, and, in assessments, or at conferences, you may be cut off before the end of your talk if you do so. In assessments, you may also be penalised.

Top tips

Telling a story

Some of the most effective and interesting presentations involve a 'story'. This could be an account of how an area of knowledge has evolved, or it could even be the story of your own research into the topic – how your knowledge and understanding developed as you surveyed the literature, and what interested or surprised you most along the way.

Organising information and ideas

Once you have selected information to be included, you need to **organise** it in the most effective manner.

- **Make it flow.** You need to structure your content in a clear, logical manner, so that it flows and is easy to follow. This will probably entail experimenting with different ways of organising what you want to say. You might find it useful to use a mind map, or to write headings and sub-headings on cards and then physically move them around.

- **Keep it simple.** Break down long segments of information into 'manageable chunks', especially if they are dense and complex. Use simple two/three/four-part organisational structures where possible. Complex content benefits from a simple organisation structure. What's more, the simpler the organisation, the easier it is for you to remember what comes next when you are delivering your presentation.

Task

What simple organisational structures could you use to structure presentations on the following topics?

1) The nursing family in the current NHS.

2) The role of nurses in palliative care.

3) Anxiety in children and young people.

Visual aids

Any visual aids such as PowerPoint slides should be of a professional standard and should be there primarily to help the audience to follow your talk, rather than simply entertaining them or, worse, bombarding them with information.

Reflection

1) What features of PowerPoint do you tend to use (think about design, colour, animations, transitions, etc)? Why do you use these features in the way you do?

2) Have you used other presentation software such as Prezi? What are the advantages and disadvantages of alternatives to PowerPoint?

The following guidelines should help you to produce slides which are an effective enhancement to your words.

Font

- Choose a font size that's visible at the back of a large room (24 pt is usually the lower limit, but it depends on the other factors – room, size of screen, etc).

- Be wary of using **bold**, *italics*, underlining or CAPITALISATION to convey subtleties of meaning as these can be hard to read on screen, especially for anyone who is dyslexic.

Colour

- Make sure there is a clear colour contrast between background and text (and remember that just because things look clear on your computer at home, it doesn't mean they will necessarily be clear on a classroom screen with different resolution and lighting conditions – always check *in situ*).

- Avoid using red and green together, as people who have a colour vision deficiency (the formal name for 'colour blindness') cannot distinguish between them.

Effects

- Avoid decorative background images that may obscure the text.

- Choose animations and transitions which are simple and effective, rather than just being there to decorate your slides or entertain.

- Be careful with moving images or flashing effects as they may be distracting or irritating – they may also be dangerous for people with epilepsy or light sensitivity.

- Make good use of the 'appear' function in PowerPoint, and practise synchronising this with your speaking: if you incorporate this feature into your slides, but then introduce all your bullet points randomly or all at once, it rather defeats the object!

- Limit the number of slides, and make sure that you are not moving through slides too quickly.

Text and images

- Make sure your slides are not cluttered with text and images.

- Limit the amount of text on the slides to 'manageable chunks', which are easily digestible.

- The text on your slides should be mostly limited to **brief prompts** (rather than full sentences) which you expand on as you speak. On slides, you can sometimes leave out 'grammar' words like verbs or words like 'a' or 'the' in a way that would not be acceptable in an essay. This is because the text on PowerPoint slides can function as a kind of shorthand. However, be careful with this if English is not your first language – it can be difficult for non-native speakers of a language to judge which grammatical words are necessary or not. If in doubt, retain the words in question.

- Do not read text verbatim from your slides. (You will bore your audience rigid and most audience members are capable of reading what's on the slides!)

- Make sure that every word, diagram and label is clearly visible, even from the back of the room. Also, make sure you have referenced those images taken from sources. (See the example slides on the following pages for examples of **Creative Commons** images, which can often be freely used without the need for acknowledgement.)

- Proofread your slides carefully to check for accuracy and consistency of formatting.

Training

- Universities often provide training on the use of PowerPoint. Check your library website for courses.

Task

Look at the following presentation slides and answer the questions.
(The notes provided after each slide provide some possible answers.)

1) How has the student used the slides to organise the presentation?

2) Are the slides clear and easy to read?

3) How has the student used diagrams to support and enhance the presentation?

BMU
British Medical University
School of Nursing and Midwifery

The nursing 'family' in healthcare

A summative presentation by
Charlotte Wei, First-Year Student Nurse

3 September 2018

The title slide always contains the title of the presentation and the name of the person doing it. It may also contain other detail such as institutional logos, the course or event the presentation is for and a date. Simple rather than fancy designs (eg black text on a white background) work best for professional presentations.

BMU
British Medical University
School of Nursing and Midwifery

Aims of the presentation

During this presentation, we will:
- explore the different types of workers within the nursing family;
- discuss what a 'nurse' is;
- explore skill mix in nursing;
- debate whether skill mix and the nursing family are good for nurses and for nursing.

It is good practice to identify some aims for your presentation. Slides generally should not be too cluttered. Any pictures or diagrams should not encroach on the copy (text) area and you should check out any copyright issues. Creative Commons images (see http://creativecommons.org) can be used freely or with simple acknowledgments. The 'bulls eye' image in the slide above is a Creative Commons 'CC0' image, which means there are no restrictions on its use, nor is any acknowledgement required.

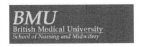

Nursing work

Four groups who do nursing work:

- healthcare/nursing assistants;
- nursing associates;
- registered nurses;
- advanced practice nurses.

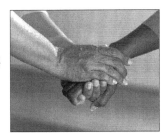

Are all of these groups nurses?

Pictures can help. The image here, like all of the images in this presentation, is also a CC0 image, so it does not need any attribution.

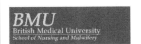

Registered nurses

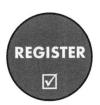

- 'Nurse' is not protected by law...
- ... but 'registered nurse' is (refers to those on the NMC Register).
- Healthcare assistants are not formally registered.
- Nursing associates will be registered by the NMC **but not as nurses**.

With bulleted lists, you might want to use some of the 'animation' options in PowerPoint to introduce each bullet in turn.

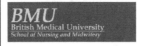

Dumbing down?

- All four groups look like nurses to the public; public doesn't know what they are getting.
- Introduction of Nursing Associate: more than a HCA; less than an RN.
- Skill mix: using fewer RNs and more HCAs/NAs puts patient safety at risk.
- 'Too posh to wash' claims about graduate RNs.

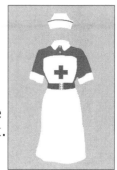

Simple images and a small amount of text work well in slides. Don't go overboard with text – some might even argue there is too much text in this slide!

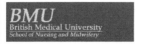

Counter-arguments

- 21st-century nursing needs RNs/ Advanced Practice Nurses (APNs).
- These are highly skilled jobs that require university degrees.
- 'Core' nursing care can be done by HCAs and Nursing Associates...
- ... so freeing RNs/APNs for higher level work: prescribing, diagnostic work, care management, etc.

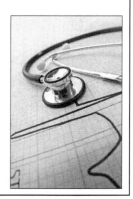

It can be useful to have discrete slides for the different sides of the argument you might be presenting.

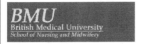

Conclusion

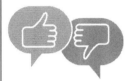

- Not everyone who does nursing is a nurse.
- The nurse of the future requires not only care and compassion, but a high level of technical and intellectual skill.
- The 'nursing family' can strengthen or dilute nursing depending on your perspective.

It's always good to have a summing up slide with a few 'headline' statements.

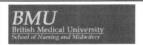

Presentation aims (revisited)

During this presentation, we have:
- explored the different types of workers within the nursing family;
- discussed what a 'nurse' is;
- explored skill mix in nursing;
- debated whether skill mix and the nursing family are good for nurses and for nursing.

Towards the end of your presentation, you might want to revisit your aims and check with the audience that you have covered them.

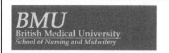

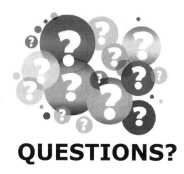

THANK YOU FOR LISTENING

QUESTIONS?

The final slide often has a 'thank you' on it and, if appropriate, a call for questions.

On the day!

As mentioned previously in the chapter, successful presentations can be delivered in a range of individual styles. As also mentioned, a lot of what happens on the day is down to your prior research and preparation, and a good understanding of context, purpose and audience. It is then a case of doing all you can to make sure that you deliver your presentation effectively on the day.

Reflection

1) How do you prepare yourself for a presentation?

2) Do you do anything to control nerves or anxiety?

3) Do you use notes during presentations? If so, how do you use them?

There are a number of useful strategies that you can adopt during your presentation to engage the audience, control nerves and make things go as smoothly as possible.

• If you are nervous before your presentation, it may help to slow your breathing or drink some water. It is OK to have water available to sip during your presentation too.

• During the presentation, address the audience directly, rather than facing the screen to read from slides or continually lowering your head to read notes. Think of a presentation as a two-way process, a conversation with the audience rather than a performance. If you engage the audience, they will communicate with you in a way through their body language, as well as through questions at the end of your presentation.

- Make eye contact with the audience, almost as you would in a conversation with someone, taking care to include as much of the room as possible. In an assessment situation, the assessors do not want you to focus on them – in fact, they will be taking note of how you establish rapport with the whole audience, how you endeavour to engage the whole room.

- Project your voice so that everyone in the room can hear you.

- Vary your intonation and pace, foregrounding and backgrounding information as required, slowing down to make something clear or to focus on a particular point; try to avoid speaking in a flat, monotone voice.

- Don't speak too quickly. It's quite common for people to speak too quickly in presentations, especially if they are nervous. Some presenters may also speak quickly to fit everything in, usually because they have not been disciplined in their selection of content! Remember also, if English is your second language, speed does not equal fluency in a language. Listen to experienced presenters and you will notice that they tend to slow down their speech on long words or when a word has particular importance. Try to do this yourself.

- Adopt a physical stance which feels relaxed and comfortable. This usually means moving around a little bit rather than standing in one place, and using your arms and hands as a natural part of communication. For example, you will probably want to physically indicate certain information on your slides at certain points.

- If you use notes, use them in a smart way. It is impressive if you can speak confidently and naturally without notes. However, many people prefer to have some notes at hand as an *aide memoire*, often written on small cards – or in the notes section of PowerPoint – just in case they get lost or forget something. This is fine – it is a good strategy to have. Just make sure you manage to look up at the audience most of the time. It is of course not a good thing to read verbatim from notes as if from an essay, or from your slides – this is extremely boring for the audience!

- Don't panic! If you lose your train of thought, pause and consult your notes or slides. Audiences are usually fairly sympathetic – they probably know how you feel!

- Practise several times to help you remember what you want to say, refine your delivery and increase your confidence. But don't learn by rote: it will sound unnatural if you try to recite something you have memorised, and straining to remember every word will make you stressed and preoccupied during the actual presentation, preventing engagement with the audience. Each practice should follow the same basic structure but there should also be some natural variation.

Top tips

Speaking well

- **Accuracy** is important, but, if English is not your first language, do not worry about making a few mistakes, as long as these do not interfere with **communication**.

- You should aim for a reasonably formal **style** – you shouldn't be too 'chatty' or vague, and you should always avoid slang.

- **Pronunciation** and **articulation** are very important. The most important thing is to be clear, and slowing down to clearly articulate key terms can help achieve this. Check the pronunciation of **key words** beforehand. Use an online dictionary with sound function (or a specialised reference work for very technical words), especially if English is not your first language. Assessors will not penalise you for having an accent (we all do!) or for the occasional mispronunciation, but they will be irritated if you keep mispronouncing a key word, and they will be unable to follow you if they cannot make out which word you are trying to say. Preparing the language you are going to use can also help you feel more in control and thus help reduce anxiety.

Top tips

Starting well!

- Greet the audience and introduce yourself, but keep it short and to the point:

  'Good morning/afternoon, my name is Gong Yi and I'm going to talk about…'

  'I am Jane Berk, from the University of Glasgow, and my main area of research is…'

- Make sure that the main subject of your talk is clearly pronounced/articulated and that it is written on the first slide.

- Try to arouse the interest of your audience with an interesting fact/anecdote/question, etc.

- Provide a clear outline of how your talk will progress – but, again, make it concise.

Ending well

- This is a chance to re-state the **main message** of your presentation in a concise, effective way. Keep it short and sweet! Be careful not to start repeating yourself in an unstructured manner.

- End the presentation cleanly and decisively – try not to waffle or repeat yourself:

'So that concludes my presentation. Thank you. Does anyone have any questions?'

Top tips

Dealing with questions

- Try to predict the most likely questions and prepare for them.

- Be prepared to reformulate questions to make sure you have understood, and to make sure the audience have also heard and understood.

- Go back to the relevant slide if necessary.

- Never have anything on your slides that you cannot explain – someone may ask you about it!

Group presentations

Group presentations present particular opportunities and challenges. They are an example of collaborative learning, something which is highly valued in universities, and many students benefit greatly from working so closely with fellow students. However, working as a group can also bring difficulties, and you will need to be prepared to address issues as they arise. Ultimately, working in a group is a learning experience in itself and you should take the opportunity to reflect on how you felt during the process and what this means for your future development (see Cartney and Rouse, 2006).

CROSS REFERENCE

Studying for your Nursing Degree, Chapter 2, Strategies for effective learning, Collaboration in action

Top tips

Working in groups

1) Agree on some basic ground rules at the beginning of the process.
2) Establish good channels of communication, either face to face or online.
3) Conduct all communication with respect and sensitivity.
4) Make the group as inclusive as possible by informing and involving everyone, and by recognising individual strengths and contributions.
5) Create an agenda for each meeting, preferably sent out beforehand so that people can prepare. During the meeting, ask for a volunteer to make notes alongside each point. You can then put these online so that everyone is clear about what has been agreed and who is responsible for any action points.

6) Encourage a constructive atmosphere where people listen to each other and acknowledge each other, negotiating respectfully and building on others' points. Give some thought to the physical arrangement of the room – is it conducive to good communication?

Poster presentations

Poster presentations are an alternative to oral presentations with slides. They are a common feature of conferences, where they can be used to present research findings, make people aware of a shared resource, or invite collaboration. For university students, they are sometimes used as a form of assessment. A student, or a group of students, will be required to create a poster which presents a summary of their research into a given topic. As with all presentations, and just as with academic writing, the purpose and audience should determine the scope and depth of the content.

Posters can be created manually, but they are usually created with bespoke software packages. These will usually be available through your library or IT website, and you may also be able to get some training on using these packages. Posters are created using both text and images (figures, graphs, tables, etc), and there are usually facilities available on campus where you can have your poster published to a professional standard, usually for a small fee.

Posters are presented in a public forum. This often resembles a type of 'market place', with people stopping to read the posters and comment or ask questions, before moving on to the next 'stall'. In this case, the poster should encourage people to engage in a dialogue about your work – though remember to also give them time to read. Alternatively, posters may stand alone without commentary. You need to consider the format of the presentation carefully when you are designing the poster, as it may well help determine the degree of explicitness required.

Posters should, above all, be clear and coherent. They should be easy to navigate, so that people can extract and process information easily. However, they also present an opportunity for you to distil complex information in a creative way.

Top tips

Creating effective posters

- Choose a title that will attract people to your poster. Short, snappy titles can be effective, as can questions (which are answered by the poster).

- Use a clear, layout, with distinct sections, headings and sub-headings. It's usually a good idea to keep things quite simple.

- Have a clear, logical flow of information. Try to imagine how the reader's eye will move over the poster. Think about how you might use features such as panels and arrows to guide them.

- Make sure all the text, including labels for figures and tables, is legible, with a font size (usually no smaller than 24 pt) that can be read at a reasonable distance.

- Keep text to a minimum, avoiding long, dense passages and making good use of concise bullet points.

- Think about how you might use diagrams, graphs and tables to present complex information in an accessible way.

- Have a good balance of text and images, and don't attempt to fill every bit of space.

- Use a limited range of colours so that the poster does not look too busy or garish. Make sure there is a clear contrast between background and text.

Peer review

It is vital to practise your presentation, and this affords an excellent opportunity to incorporate peer review into your practice. Some assessment tasks may also take account of feedback from your peers. When conducting peer reviews in practice sessions, it is a good idea to put together a feedback sheet like the one in Figure 3.1 to use to review each other's presentations, as this will both help you to give useful feedback to your fellow students and encourage you to reflect on how you can improve your own performance.

SPEAKER: TOPIC:	YES/NO	NOTES/ COMMENTS
1) Were you able to follow the general gist of the presentation?		
2) Was the information clearly and logically organised?		
3) Was there an appropriate amount of detail?		
4) Were specialist concepts and terminology adequately defined and explained?		
5) Did the slides help you to understand the topic and follow the line of argument?		
6) Were any words/phrases hard to catch because they were said too quickly or mispronounced?		
7) Did the presenter engage you as an audience member? How? How could they have done this more?		
8) Did the presenter keep to time?		

Figure 3.1: Example peer review sheet

Being assessment literate

Presentations, both individual presentations and group presentations, are a common form of assessment. As with any assessment, it is important to inform yourself of what is required and how you will be assessed. This is sometimes referred to as being '**assessment literate**' (Price et al, 2012). You can become assessment literate by paying close attention to the **wording of the task**, and by familiarising yourself with both the **assessment guidelines** and the **marking descriptors** for the task. Lecturers themselves will refer closely to these when assessing your presentation, so it is very important that you pay close attention to them throughout the planning and practice stages of your presentation.

Below are some example presentation tasks at levels 4, 5 and 6, followed by a table containing marking descriptors which distinguish between what is expected at the three levels (4, 5, 6) of your undergraduate degree.

CROSS
REFERENCE

Appendix 1,
Academic
levels at
university

Example assessment tasks

1) Present to your seminar group a 20-minute presentation on: 'Activities of Daily Living' (level 4).

2) In groups of four to five, deliver a 15-minute presentation on: 'Anxiety in Children and Young People' (level 4).

3) In a 20-minute presentation (including question time), answer the question 'Is mindfulness a useful tool for nursing practice?' (level 5).

4) Deliver a group presentation on the evidence-base for restricting visiting times in hospitals. You will have 15 minutes to present and 5 minutes for questions (level 5).

5) In a 20-minute presentation (including question time), critically outline how you would lead and implement change in a clinical area relevant to your field of practice (level 6).

6) 'Nurses are the ideal professionals to lead on health promotion.' Critically explore this statement in a 20-minute group presentation with four to five of your peers (level 6).

Table 3.1: Example presentation marking descriptors

Level 4
• Demonstrates knowledge and understanding of the topic area.
• Provides clear slides or other visual prompts that are accessible by all, including those with a disability.
• Demonstrates good verbal and non-verbal communication skills (tone of voice, body language, demeanour, etc).

- Keeps to time and paces the presentation well.
- (For group presentations) Demonstrates reasonable rapport with fellow presenters.

Level 5
- Demonstrates critical understanding of the topic area by providing arguments for and against.
- Provides clear slides or other visual prompts that are accessible by all, including those with a disability.
- Demonstrates good verbal and non-verbal communication skills (tone of voice, body language, demeanour, etc).
- Keeps to time and paces the presentation well.
- Responds to questions posed by the audience confidently.
- (For group presentations) Demonstrates rapport with fellow presenters.
- (For group presentations) Transitions to fellow presenters are good.

Level 6
- Demonstrates critical evaluation of the topic area by making reference to the evidence base.
- Shows emerging evidence of originality in the arguments made.
- Provides clear slides or other visual prompts that are accessible by all, including those with a disability.
- Demonstrates a high level of verbal and non-verbal communication skills (tone of voice, body language, demeanour, etc).
- Keeps to time and paces the presentation well.
- Responds to questions posed by the audience confidently.
- (For group presentations) Clear evidence of rapport with, and seamless transitions between, fellow presenters.

Task

1) Look at the assessment tasks and marking descriptors laid out above. What are the main differences between levels in terms of what is expected from students? What particular phrases in the presentation tasks and marking descriptors tell you this?

2) Brainstorm some ideas for each of the presentation tasks. Which of the tasks seem most interesting to you? Why? Which seem most difficult? Why?

3) Which of the descriptors do you think present the biggest challenges for you as you develop as an academic presenter?

Advanced skills

Three minute thesis

When you are at the stage of writing a dissertation, or even conducting postgraduate research, you will need to present your research to various audiences. When you are deep into a research topic, it can be difficult to shift your perspective to match that of people who have not been on your particular research journey. Many presenters can get bogged down in the detail of their research and ultimately fail to convey the essence of their topic. It could help you to avoid this pitfall if you have a look at some of the entries to the **three minute thesis** competition founded by the University of Queensland in 2008. The idea for the competition originated in a slightly unusual way:

'The idea for the 3MT competition came about at a time when the state of Queensland was suffering severe drought. To conserve water, residents were encouraged to time their showers, and many people had a three minute egg timer fixed to the wall in their bathroom. The then Dean of the UQ Graduate School, Emeritus Professor Alan Lawson, put two and two together and the idea for the 3MT competition was born.'

Students entering the competition are required to 'effectively explain their research in three minutes, in a language appropriate to a non-specialist audience', using only one slide. Many universities invite their students to take part in the competition, and most have a web page with videos of some of the best entries. Watching some of these may give you an idea of how to identify the essential components of your research topic and to distil them into something which an audience can easily process and fully appreciate.

Summary

This chapter has explored the nature and challenges of public speaking, with a focus on the types of academic presentation which are likely to be a requirement of your degree programme. It has provided strategies for preparing and delivering presentations, both as an individual and in groups, in an effective, engaging way, focusing on content, organisation, visual aids and delivery. It has also provided examples of tasks at different levels of your degree programmes, along with example descriptors which show what is expected of you at each level.

References

Cartney, P and Rouse, A (2006) The Emotional Impact of Learning in Small Groups: Highlighting the Impact on Student Progression and Retention. *Teaching in Higher Education*, 111(1): 79–81.

Mercer, N, Warwick, P and Ahmed, A (2017) An Oracy Assessment Toolkit: Linking Research and Development in the Assessment of Students' Spoken Language Skills at Age 11–12. *Learning and Instruction*, 48: 51–60.

Price, M, Rust, C, O'Donovan, B and Handley, K (2012) *Assessment Literacy: The Foundation for Improving Student Learning*. Oxford: Oxford Brookes University Press.

Three Minute Thesis, University of Queensland [online]. Available at: https://threeminutethesis.uq.edu.au/home (accessed 23 October 2018).

Chapter 4
Participating in group seminars and meetings

Learning outcomes

After reading this chapter you will:

- be better prepared to participate in group discussion;

- have a good understanding of the role that group discussion and seminars play both in your studies and in your intellectual development;

- be aware of the transferable nature of seminar skills;

- be able to participate more fully and confidently in group discussions, seminars and meetings in academic and professional life;

- have explored strategies to help you participate more effectively in group discussions, seminars and meetings, and to get more from them.

This chapter looks at the topic of group discussion, particularly in the form of seminars. It explores the role seminars play in your university studies, and it familiarises you with certain conventions and language which are important in a seminar setting. This knowledge will help you to participate more fully in seminars. You will also develop an understanding of how the skills you develop in seminars can transfer to your professional life, and help you in teamwork activities and meetings.

The role of seminars at university

Group discussion is an important part of university life, and seminars are the main type of group discussion at university. Seminars usually involve relatively small numbers of students, usually around 8 to 12, but this can vary across institutions and courses. You may or may not have participated in seminars previously, but before reading more about them in this chapter, take some time to reflect on what you think might be the aims and outcomes of seminars.

Task

---

1) What do you think is the purpose of a seminar?

2) Below are some statements about seminars. Did you think of any of these when answering question 1?

a) Seminars provide an opportunity to follow up on a lecture. They allow you to explore and demonstrate your understanding of the topic, and to clarify anything that you didn't understand from the lecture itself.

b) Seminar discussion can enable you to forge a deeper understanding of ideas and concepts.

c) Seminar discussions can be good preparation for essays, exams and other assessments, as they provide a space for you to test your understanding and ideas, and work out how to express them in a clear, convincing way.

d) Seminars provide an opportunity to learn from people with different knowledge, background, experience and perspectives from your own.

e) Seminar discussion may lead you to change, develop or adapt your opinions and ideas as you come into contact with others' views.

f) Some seminar activities can help you develop your problem-solving skills.

g) Frequent participation in seminars can help you become more confident about public speaking.

h) Seminars can help you become more confident about discussing complex issues and ideas.

i) Seminars can help you improve the way you interact with others in a group setting.

j) Seminar skills are transferable skills which can help you in your professional practice, for example in teamwork and meetings with colleagues.

3) Which of the things mentioned in the statements above do you think are most important for you as a university student?

4) Which of the statements do you think refer to:
- developing your **communication** skills;
- developing your **thinking**;
- both of these?

As the statements in the task explain, seminars can be used to develop or test your understanding of a topic. On some courses they are used as a form of **assessment**, testing both your knowledge of a topic and your ability to interact successfully in a group discussion. Below, there are some examples of typical seminar tasks at different levels, with an indication of how they would be assessed.

CROSS REFERENCE

Appendix 1, Academic levels at university

Example seminar tasks and assessment criteria

Example 1 (level 4)

'You were given a paper to read on the history of nursing for this week's seminar. Based on your reading of this paper (and any other materials you may have read), together with your direct experience of nursing so far, discuss with your seminar group colleagues the statement "nursing was better in the past than it is now".'

If the seminar is assessed, a student's engagement in the seminar might be judged according to the following criteria:

- *Provided evidence that they have read the paper beforehand.*
- *Made a positive contribution to the group.*
- *Provided strong arguments for or against nursing being better in the past than it is now.*
- *Acted in a professional and courteous manner when interacting with others.*

Example 2 (level 5)

'In small groups, spend 10–15 minutes critically exploring the role that Mental Health Nurses can play in:

- integrating mental and physical health in the general population
- promoting mental health and preventing mental ill-health (rather than treating mental illness).'

If the seminar is assessed, a student's engagement in the seminar might be judged according to the following criteria:

- *Made a positive contribution to the group.*
- *Provided examples of how Mental Health Nurses might integrate mental and physical health and/or promote mental health and prevent mental ill-health.*
- *Provided evidence of critical ability (eg challenging others' views, offering alternative stances, referring to the evidence-base).*
- *Acted in a professional and courteous manner when interacting with others.*

Example 3 (level 6)

'With your seminar group colleagues, pick one of the three case scenarios that were published to the group last week and provide a care plan for the patient/ service user at the centre of the scenario.'

If the seminar is assessed, a student's engagement in the seminar might be judged according to the following criteria:

- *Contributed to the group choice of case scenario.*
- *Provided strong evidence for the use (or not, as the case may be) for a particular nursing model.*
- *Demonstrated critical use of the nursing process (or other problem-solving approach).*
- *Contributed to the evidence-base for the care plan.*
- *Acted in a professional and courteous manner when interacting with others.*
- *Demonstrated leadership skills (eg actively facilitates discussion, encourages others to speak, actively listens to others).*

The conventions of seminars

Like all community activities, seminars are governed by certain conventions of behaviour. All conventions are determined by the norms, values and practices of the community in question, in this case the academic community. Seminar conventions are intended to facilitate discussion, promote academic activity and development, and help the people involved feel comfortable and engaged.

Reflection

Look at some of the conventions associated with successful seminar participation below:

- Preparing before the seminar;
- Turn taking;
- Making a contribution to the discussion;
- Making eye contact with the whole group when you speak;
- Backing up your ideas and arguments with clear explanation and reasoning;
- Supporting your ideas and arguments with evidence and examples where possible;
- Reformulating what you have said if others appear not to understand;
- Acknowledging others' contributions and building on them;
- Paying attention to others when they are speaking and listening carefully to what they have to say;
- Asking for clarification when you haven't understood somebody else's point;
- Expressing agreement;
- Expressing cautious agreement;
- Expressing polite disagreement;
- Challenging others' ideas and arguments when you think they are wrong or unclear;
- Interrupting politely;
- Inviting others to participate;
- Reaching a consensus (particularly with problem-solving activities);
- Summing up the discussion.

1) Why do you think these things are considered to be important?
2) Can you think of examples which demonstrate their importance?
3) How do they relate to the requirements of the assessments in the previous section to be 'professional' and 'courteous' in interaction with others?
4) Which ones could relate to the 'leadership' requirements of the assessments (facilitating discussion, encouraging others to speak, actively listening to others)?

Task

Look at the extracts from student seminars below. Which of the conventions in the previous reflection task are they related to?

1) 'Wouldn't you say that poverty is a factor here?'

2) 'Yes, but what about parity of esteem between mental and physical health?'

3) 'But surely that's the role of government?'

4) 'What do you think Claire?'

5) 'As Mia said, the policy seems to disadvantage family carers and advantage the government, who essentially get care from relatives free of charge.'

6) 'I think Portugal is a good example of somewhere where drug addiction is seen as a health issue rather than a criminal issue.'

7) 'Did you say you worked with people with dementia on your placement, Lia?'

8) 'Could I just add something to what Dan said?'

9) 'Aren't we forgetting the impact of peer pressure?"

10) 'But isn't that more an issue of compliance? Or is it "concordance" or "adherence" that we use now?'

11) 'I take your point, but what about patient autonomy?'

12) 'I see what you mean, but why is that important?'

13) 'According to one of the studies we were asked to look at, there is some evidence to suggest that the treatment can be effective if it is combined with other therapies.'

14) 'But didn't that study have a really small sample size?'

15) 'I didn't quite catch what you said about the stats.'

16) 'Sorry, could you just explain what you mean by "alternative therapies"? I ask because lots of different therapies with widely varying evidence bases get lumped together under that heading.'

17) 'I'm afraid I don't quite follow your point.'

18) 'So what you're saying is that we need to provide different types of support.'

19) 'Yes, that's a really good example.'

20) 'Yes, I hadn't thought of that.'

21) 'Are you sure about that? It's not how I interpreted it.'

22) 'I don't really think that what you're suggesting is realistic, given the current financial crisis in the NHS.'

23) 'Are we all agreed on that?'

Participating effectively in seminars

In order to participate effectively in seminars, it is important to be aware of the conventions discussed in the previous section, understand why they are important and be willing to adhere to them wherever possible. Some of these conventions will be discussed in more detail in the following sections.

Being prepared

You may be asked to read some material before the seminar, for example, a research article or some case studies. One or two students may be asked to lead the seminar by summarising and commenting on the reading material, leading to a wider group discussion. Preparation could also involve researching different views and perspectives on a topic.

Good preparation should enable you to participate in the seminar. And if you are indeed well prepared, it is a pity to waste all that work by staying silent! If you do not contribute during the seminar, it may signal a lack of preparation or engagement, which will not be appreciated by your lecturers or fellow students, and which could lead to poor marks if you are being assessed.

On the other hand, whereas good preparation is essential, and it is clearly good to have an idea of what you are going to say during the seminar, try not to be too 'rehearsed'. A seminar should promote natural dialogue rather than generate formal speeches.

Top tips

Summarising articles

You can use certain verbs to help you structure your article summary.

1) Giving an overview

The article The author	deals with examines discusses reports on argues that found (that)

2) Indicating the structure of the article

The article The author	begins/starts by _____ing goes on to… then… ends/finishes by _____ing concludes that…

3) Identifying strengths and weaknesses of the article

The article The author	was interesting in that it… puts forward a strong argument in favour of… identifies the probable cause of… did not address… fails to mention… confuses the issue, in my view…

Helping to construct meaning

Seminars are an opportunity to create and explore ideas as a group in a way that would perhaps not be possible on an individual level. Ideally, the ideas discussed are 'emergent and co-constructed', rather than 'presented as already formed for inspection' (Alexander et al, 2011, p 237). People in the group work together to make sense of the issues, ideas, data, etc and are therefore ultimately able to establish better understanding and deeper meaning. You will take your individual thoughts and ideas (and doubts) into the seminar, just as others bring their own thoughts and ideas (and doubts). What is expected is that interaction and collaboration will lead to an interesting synthesis of ideas, and that this will allow individuals to reach conclusions that they could not have reached alone in their room with their lecture notes and books.

Interacting with the group

Successful group interaction is dependent on a number of factors. These are centred around:

- being fully engaged and encouraging others to be fully engaged;
- feeling respected and respecting each other;
- feeling comfortable and making others feel comfortable.

This involves the following.

CROSS REFERENCE

Chapter 1, Professional speaking skills, Active listening

- **Speaking**. It is important that all members of the group make a contribution of some kind. Your individual contribution will vary according to the day or the topic. Sometimes, you may make a significant contribution because you feel confident that you are in full command of the study material or you feel passionate about the topic. Other times, you may make a smaller contribution. This may even just involve responding to another student's contribution, but this in itself can be important. Note that complete silence denotes a lack of involvement and engagement, which is not good for you or for the group. For some people, it can be a bit nerve-wracking to speak for the first time in front of a group, but try to reassure yourself that the second time will almost undoubtedly be easier. Most universities keep students in the same seminar groups for a period of time so that supportive relationships can develop.

- **Listening**. Good listening skills are as important as good speaking skills. The way you respond to someone else's ideas contributes to the general discussion. Your responses are a way of showing that you are fully engaged and paying close attention to what other people are saying. How you respond can also say as much about your intellectual abilities as does your expression of your own ideas, which is particularly important if the seminar task is being assessed.

- **Body language**. There are a number of things which people sometimes do without thinking, and even though the people who do these things may not mean any disrespect, their actions may signal a lack of interest and engagement, or imply that they are not taking the seminar seriously. These include: looking down or away when someone is talking, checking phones, eye rolling, sighing or tutting.

CROSS REFERENCE

Participating in group seminars and meetings, Mind your language

- **Being assertive without being rude**. This can be tricky to navigate, but it is essential to bear it in mind. While it is important to be able to say what you think in a confident way, and to be able to disagree with others when necessary, it is also crucial that you do this without upsetting people or causing the discussion to become strained. Politeness is related to the words you use, the tone of your voice, and your body language. Polite language use will be discussed later in the chapter.

- **Turn taking**. It is important to take turns in a way which ensures everybody is given the opportunity to speak, and no one person dominates the discussion. Turns can be long or short, ranging from leading the seminar, to putting forward a fairly detailed argument, to responding briefly to someone else's contribution. Those who facilitate seminars (lecturers and sometime students themselves) will often ensure that everyone gets a chance to speak, encouraging the quieter students to speak and more assertive ones to hold back a little.

- **Negotiating**. Negotiation is a part of the co-construction of meaning. It is part of the to-and-fro of dynamic discussion, of working out the facts and deciding what they mean. It involves asserting and questioning, confirming and clarifying, and agreeing and disagreeing. Negotiation is also a necessary part of organising and facilitating group interaction. This may involve deciding how to proceed at a particular part of the discussion – eg whether to move on to the next topic, summarise the discussion so far, or perhaps even take a vote.

CROSS REFERENCE

Participating in group seminars and meetings, Helping to construct meaning

- **Giving and eliciting confirmation and clarification**. As mentioned in the previous point, this forms part of the negotiation and co-construction of meaning. Confirming what you meant by something or asking someone else what they meant by something is an important part of discussion, as is providing or asking for clarification. These things help ensure that people do not reach conclusions based on a lack of information or on misunderstanding.

CROSS REFERENCE

Academic Writing and Referencing for your Nursing Degree, Chapter 3, Referring to sources

- **Acknowledging others' ideas**. The importance of this is often underestimated in seminars. In academia, it is essential that contributions to a field are fully acknowledged. Similarly, in a seminar or other group discussion, it is important to acknowledge how what you say repeats or builds on what someone else has said, using phrases such as 'As Annie said…' or 'Just to add to what Paul was saying about patient autonomy…'. This is important in a seminar for two reasons: 1) It reflects the value academia places on source attribution and avoidance of plagiarism; 2) It facilitates the flow of a discussion: if people repeat the same idea or a similar idea without signalling that it repeats or relates closely to what someone else has said, the discussion can become static and fragmented; acknowledging how ideas are connected and build on each other contributes to the smooth flow of the discussion.

- **Setting some ground rules**. If you do this at the beginning of the process – in your first seminar meeting with a particular group – it can help facilitate group interaction and avoid friction. The following **case study** relating the experiences of a university lecturer illustrates the point.

Case study

There are some students who always come late to seminars or don't do the preparatory work beforehand. This irritates other students who have, on many occasions, waited for the seminar to end so they can complain directly to me about this behaviour in the hope that I will confront these 'wayward' students. When I explain that the philosophy behind group work in seminars is such that students should challenge each other over unacceptable behaviour rather than depend on a lecturer to discipline and control, the students often say that they don't like challenging their peers, especially if they otherwise get on with them! I have given tips about how to broach the subject using such phrases as 'I'm sorry, this is nothing personal but we're supposed to be working as a group so it's important we all do what we're supposed to do'. Setting clear ground rules beforehand can help, as can reminding students that dealing with difficult situations (and people) is an inherent part of nursing practice so it is something they have to get used to.

Transferable skills

Seminar skills are important if you are to participate effectively in seminars – this goes without saying. However, it is also important to understand that many of the skills you develop in seminars are transferrable, ie useful in other areas of life, in particular, in your professional practice. These transferable skills include:

- meeting skills (eg interaction, turn taking, reaching a consensus, polite disagreement);
- intellectual skills (criticality, creativity);
- communication skills;
- linguistic skills;
- collaborative skills;
- social skills;
- intercultural skills.

These skills are important skills as far as the NMC Code (2015) is concerned in that they underpin a great deal of the Code's core elements, including Section 7 (communicating clearly), Sections 8 and 9 (working cooperatively and sharing skills and knowledge), Section 17 (raising concerns), Section 19 (reducing risks of harm), Section 23 (cooperating with investigations) and Section 25 (providing leadership).

Meetings in a professional setting

As a nurse, you will be required to attend, and indeed facilitate, many different types of meeting. These could be staff meetings, ward rounds, therapeutic meetings (eg group work in mental health) where you lead as the therapist, disciplinary meetings (hopefully as a panel member and not as the person being disciplined!), case conferences and various types of committee. The skills required for these meetings are similar to those required for seminars, eg listening to the viewpoints of others and putting yours across assertively, being polite and diplomatic in your demeanour, sharing appropriate information and helping negotiate solutions to problems.

Mind your language

We all know that, in many situations, it's not what we say, but how we say it that counts. Notions of acceptable interaction can be different among different individuals and different cultures. Some individuals are more direct than others and may even come across as quite blunt; others are less direct and more circumspect in their interactions, and may even come across as lacking in assertiveness. Similarly, patterns of interaction which are acceptable in one culture may not be acceptable in another.

Case studies

A

While running a workshop on seminar skills, I was approached by a lecturer from overseas who was distraught by the fact that she seemed to be upsetting some students in her seminars. After some discussion, it became apparent that the lecturer would ask a question, and, if the answer was not what she was looking for, she would simply say 'no' and ask someone else. This had appeared to make some students uncomfortable, but she had no idea why, as this way of interacting had been perfectly acceptable in her home university. I explained that British people are generally more comfortable with less direct responses, particularly in a group situation where they might feel under scrutiny. We discussed the use of typical expressions we might use in this situation in order to 'soften' or 'cushion' what we say, such as 'I think I see what you mean but…', 'I take your point but…', 'I'm not quite sure that really addresses the point…'. The lecturer was surprised by this indirect approach as it did not match the conventions of her own culture, which allowed for a more direct approach, but she was nevertheless keen to try out the phrases in class as her main concern was that students should feel they were in a comfortable learning environment.

B

I was teaching a group of Mongolian students on an academic skills course. One of the main activities was a seminar. I was extremely impressed with the amount of preparation they had done and with the quality of their contributions. In particular, I noticed that they had all used really interesting examples from the media to support their arguments. I mentioned this later, while giving general feedback to the group. They nodded eagerly when I mentioned the quality of the examples, but I had noticed that they hadn't seemed very impressed at the time – in fact, they had not reacted at all to each other's examples. So I asked the students if they had considered commenting positively during the seminar, by saying, for instance, 'I think that's a really good example'. They all laughed a little and explained that this felt a bit strange: 'We just wouldn't do that.' However, they did agree to give it a go in the next seminar.

Task

Softening your language

1) Here are some phrases from earlier in the chapter. Find the words or phrases in each group that 'soften' the students' contributions.

A

'Wouldn't you say that social class is a factor here?'

'Aren't we forgetting the impact of peer pressure?'

'But wasn't that a really small study?'

'That's doubtful, isn't it?'

B

'Yes, but what about the wider issues?'

'I take your point, but what about patient autonomy?'

'I see what you mean, but why is that important?'

C

'Could I just add something to what Dan said?'

'Sorry, could you just explain what you mean by "alternative therapies"?'

'I didn't quite catch what you said about the stats.'

'I'm afraid I don't quite follow your point.'

'I don't really think that what you're suggesting is realistic, given the current financial crisis in the NHS.'

2) Match each group (A, B, C) to the correct explanation (i, ii, iii).

i) Some 'little' words like 'just', 'quite' and 'really' are often used to soften or cushion a request, comment or criticism. In some of these cases, the use of 'sorry' or 'I'm afraid' further softens the intervention.

ii) The 'negative' question form can seem less direct or challenging than a direct question form. Question tags like 'isn't it?' can also have the same effect. Tone of voice and intonation are also factors here.

iii) Some 'yes, but…' structures, sometimes called 'pivot' structures, can cushion a disagreement, as they serve to acknowledge the validity of the other person's opinion before begging to differ.

Top tips

Softening your language: a summary

Negative questions (these usually have 'not' in them in their abbreviated form '…n't'):

- 'Wouldn't you say…?'
- 'Don't you think…?'
- 'Aren't we forgetting…?'

'Pivot' expressions (note key use of 'but'):

- 'I see what you mean but…'
- 'I think I understand where you're coming from but…'
- 'I take your point but…'

Little words ('just', 'quite', 'really'):

- 'Can I just say that…'
- 'Could you just explain what you mean by…'
- 'I don't quite follow.'
- 'That's not quite what I mean.'
- 'I don't really understand what you mean.'
- 'That's not really relevant.'

Summary

This chapter has explored the skills you need to participate effectively in group discussions, including seminars and meetings. It has discussed the role seminars play in your university studies, and introduced conventions and language which are important in a seminar setting. It has also looked at how the skills you develop in seminars can transfer to your professional life, eg the teamwork activities and meetings you might have to engage in as a registered health professional.

References

Alexander, A, Argent, S and Spencer, J (2011) *EAP Essentials: A Teacher's Guide to Principles and Practice*. Reading: Garnet Publishing Ltd.

NMC (Nursing and Midwifery Council) (2015) *The Code: Professional Standards of Practice and Behaviour for Nurses and Midwives* [online]. Available at: www.nmc.org.uk/globalassets/sitedocuments/nmc-publications/nmc-code.pdf (accessed 2 September 2018).

Chapter 5
Getting the most from individual tutorials

Learning outcomes

After reading this chapter you will:

- have a good understanding of the role of tutorials in your studies;

- be better aware of the 'etiquette' of tutorials;

- have explored strategies which can help you to make the most of tutorials.

This chapter will help you to understand the role tutorials play in your academic studies and become better aware of the 'etiquette' associated with them. It will also provide you with strategies that can help you to make the most of this valuable, but usually very limited, time with your lecturers and advisers.

What is a tutorial?

A tutorial is a meeting with an academic member of staff. The Quality Assurance Agency for Higher Education (QAA) defines it as: 'a meeting involving one-to-one or small group supervision, feedback or detailed discussion on a particular topic or project' (2011, p 6). This could be with a **lecturer** on a particular module, including the **module leader**, or it could with be your **personal tutor**, a member of academic staff assigned to provide you with guidance and support.

In most universities, a tutorial is normally a one-to-one meeting, in contrast with a lecture or a seminar, where larger groups of students are present. (Indeed, in lectures, sometimes hundreds of students may be present.) Occasionally, however, there may be more than one student present – maybe two or three. In fact, in some universities, a tutorial can be synonymous with a seminar, a small discussion group. However, the QAA (2011, p 15) distinguishes tutorials from seminars in terms of 'the stronger emphasis they place on the role of the tutor in giving direction and feedback'. This differentiation is important because it tells you what you should expect from a tutorial: not just advice and guidance but, specifically, **direction and feedback**.

CROSS REFERENCE

Chapter 4, Participating in group seminars and meetings

Tutorials are usually face-to-face meetings, though occasionally they are conducted over the phone or through some virtual meeting software like Skype rather than in person. Telephone tutorials are often more convenient than virtual meetings, as the latter require a stable, fast internet connection. However, virtual meeting software with video function has the advantage of retaining the nuances of body language present in most face-to-face meetings.

Tutorials may be scheduled as part of your timetable, with each student being given a particular time slot to meet with their lecturers or personal tutors. Many lecturers have **office hours** where they meet students, usually on a one-to-one basis. Depending on the institution, department or individual lecturer, you may need to email to book a tutorial, or there may be an open 'drop-in' session, where lecturers deal with queries on a first-come-first-served basis.

It is a good idea to find out about the conventions for tutorials at the beginning of your studies. Universities are adult learning environments which promote individual student responsibility, so you might have to initiate a request for a tutorial rather than wait for your lecturer or personal tutor to contact you. You should be able to find guidelines on tutorials in your course handbook or module guide, or on your Virtual Learning Environment (VLE) – usually Blackboard or Moodle. Most lecturers will be quite flexible about meeting you individually if you email them to arrange an appointment – just try to give plenty of notice and an indication of flexible availability, and be aware of particularly busy times of year for lecturers, such as periods of marking immediately after exams.

Why do you have tutorials at university?

Tutorials, particularly one-to-one tutorials, are a valuable opportunity for individual contact time with a member of academic staff. They are a chance to speak to a lecturer or personal tutor about a number of possible issues, including:

- your academic progress;
- concepts and skills important to your studies;
- learning how to make good study and research choices;
- learning how to think, study and research independently;
- the mark and feedback you've received in a particular assignment;
- pastoral issues, ie your individual development and welfare.

Tutorials with a module lecturer are usually concerned with academic issues; tutorials with a personal tutor may address both academic and personal issues.

Tutorials provide important individual support with your studies. As the QAA states (2011, p 6), an individual tutorial is probably the best chance you will have to gain personalised '**direction and feedback**', and these can have a significant effect on your academic attainment. Lecturer **direction** could relate to an area of your studies which you have found particularly difficult to understand, or a particular skill which you need to work on. Individual **feedback** from your lecturers is something which is essential to progress in all areas of academic life, including academic writing and speaking, and all areas of your nursing studies, including your reflective portfolio or the development of your clinical skills.

Having a tutorial is especially important if you have failed a particular piece of work, since the direction and feedback in these circumstances is normally designed to be remedial, that is, to help you succeed on a further attempt. You might also arrange an academic writing tutorial in this case (discussed in the next section).

Academic writing tutorials

Most universities provide one-to-one **academic writing tutorials**, sometimes known as **academic writing consultations**. This is an opportunity to meet with an expert in English language and academic skills to discuss a piece of your writing – either something still in progress or something you've already received feedback on from a nursing lecturer.

In the case of a piece of work in progress, the tutor will be able to provide advice on how to improve it before submission. Note that these tutorials do not constitute a proofreading service. Some of the discussion will relate directly to the piece of work in question – how you might improve organisation, grammar, punctuation, style or word choice – but the main aim is to provide information and advice which you can apply more generally, helping you to develop into a better academic writer. This might involve thinking about how to plan and organise ideas in a coherent way, or how to link ideas together to form cohesive paragraphs. Proofreading is a more mechanical process, usually involving checking grammar and punctuation at the surface level of text at the very end of the writing process. This would simply not be the best use of the writing tutor's expertise.

In the case of a piece of work that has already been marked, the tutor will be able to help you understand the mark and the feedback you received. For example, a lecturer's comment to 'use a more academic style' may be more concretely explained as 'here you should have avoided the word "get" – better to use "obtain" instead', or 'personal pronouns are essential in a reflective essay, but a critical or theoretical essay tends to be more impersonal in tone, so it's best to avoid phrases like "I think we should" – try using phrases like "there is a strong argument for" when giving your opinion'.

The fact that a writing tutor is not an expert in nursing can be very beneficial for you, as they can tell you if your explanations of nursing concepts and theories are largely understandable (excluding very technical detail) to a general audience, as they should be. In this sense, the tutor assumes the role of a 'critical friend'.

Students are usually restricted to one tutorial per semester, or even one per year, so make sure that you use the opportunity well. An academic writing tutorial is not a silver bullet. It will not solve all your writing problems or turn you into a better writer overnight. Developing as a writer is an incremental process based on a cycle of practice and feedback from a range of academic staff over time. But a writing tutorial can kick-start the process in many cases. In our experience, for many students, it can be a 'light-bulb' moment when they begin to understand where they were perhaps going wrong, and what simple steps they can take to make noticeable improvements. However, you need to be open to discussing your work critically if you are to benefit. If you are overly defensive about what you have written, it will be difficult to move forward. Remember, you are trying to write for a *reader* (the lecturer who marks your work or the writing tutor, both of whom have experience of reading hundreds of essays every year), and this is a rare but

CROSS REFERENCE

Academic Writing and Referencing for your Nursing Degree, Chapter 1, Academic writing: text, process and criticality; Chapter 2, Coherent texts and arguments

CROSS REFERENCE

Academic Writing and Referencing for your Nursing Degree, Chapter 5, Preparing your work for submission, Editing and proofreading your final text

CROSS REFERENCE

Academic Writing and Referencing for your Nursing Degree, Chapter 4, Language in use invaluable opportunity to talk to that reader about their actual experience when reading your work.

Personal tutors

The role of a personal tutor varies across institutions, faculties and schools. However, all personal tutors in some way act as a gateway to the wider institution. They will point you in the direction of the wide variety of student support and development services that most universities provide, so they should be the first person you contact if you feel you need extra support or training. Examples of the types of support and development services UK universities provide include:

- in-sessional support in English language, mainly directed at international students, eg grammar workshops or pronunciation classes;
- in-sessional support in academic skills focusing on areas such as academic reading (eg reading journal articles), academic writing (eg writing essays), academic listening (eg note taking in lectures) and academic speaking (eg giving academic presentations or participating in seminars); this support may be directed at international students, but it is increasingly open to all students;
- academic writing tutorials;
- disability support;
- financial, housing and social support;
- counselling.

Personal tutors are normally the first choice in providing you with references for future study or employment, although other lecturers may also be able to do this.

Tutorials in nursing

Since nursing is a practice-based discipline, discussions of clinical practice often feature in tutorials on nursing courses. These discussions can take many forms (as you will see in the following case studies) and include:

CROSS REFERENCE

Critical Thinking for your Nursing Degree, Chapter 2, Reflective practice

- discussions with a module lecturer as to how you might apply theory to your field of nursing practice for an assignment;
- discussions with your personal tutor about difficulties you are having with a particular placement;
- discussions with either module lecturers or personal tutors about the role of reflection in enhancing your own nursing practice;
- practical discussions about the organisation of health or care services in your local area.

Case studies

Look at the case studies below. What might the students do in each case? How might they benefit from speaking to a lecturer or personal tutor in a one-to-one tutorial?

A

Sandra has had feedback on an essay which has caused her some concern. She worked very hard on the essay, but even though the feedback indicated that most of the content was relevant, it also stated that she needed to improve her academic writing skills. However, it doesn't really go into much detail, and she's not really sure what she's doing wrong. She has seen that the university runs a number of courses on academic writing, but she thinks these may be aimed at foreign students who don't speak English as a first language and need help with grammar (Sandra was born and educated in Leeds).

B

Paulo's grandmother is very sick and has not been given long to live. She is back in his home town in Brazil, but he is not sure if he will be able to get back to see her. He has always been very close to her and is feeling extremely upset. He is not able to focus on his studies at all.

C

Laila's practice supervisor has been in touch with Laila's personal tutor saying that Laila hasn't been turning up for her placements and that, on the occasions she has turned up, she is often late. Laila's personal tutor asks to see her.

D

Mark is concerned that a couple of popular students in his peer group have been posting material on social media that he feels is incompatible with the NMC Code. However, he is worried that there might be repercussions if he reports them, eg that the rest of the group might ostracise him or call him a troublemaker, or that he might be jeopardising someone's future career by reporting them.

E

Shazia overheard a patient refer to her using a racist term. She's upset about this, particularly as the patient had always appeared pleasant to her. The patient had not said anything offensive directly to her; she had just heard it while she was in the next cubicle. She later mentioned this to the ward manager, who told her it was 'just part of the job' and she should 'toughen up'. This has made Shazia think about leaving nursing despite the fact that it has always been her dream job.

Discussion of case studies

A

Many students struggle with academic writing, so it is important not to be embarrassed or bury your head in the sand. Sandra may be right that the academic writing courses on offer are aimed at international students, but in fact, most universities have come to realise that *all* students can have issues with academic writing, regardless of their background, and these universities are increasingly making academic writing courses more widely available. It is also true that universities often provide classes to help international students with grammar, but academic writing courses usually deal with much wider issues, such as structuring an essay, developing a clear argument, and making appropriate reference to sources. Furthermore, it is not just international students who can benefit from polishing their grammar and punctuation! If Sandra has a one-to-one tutorial with the lecturer who marked the essay, they will be able to be more specific about which aspects of her writing need attention, and they will probably reassure her that she is not the only student dealing with these issues. Both lecturers and personal tutors will be able to provide more information on in-sessional writing courses or individual academic writing tutorials that the university provides.

CROSS
REFERENCE

Academic
writing
tutorials

B

In the first instance, Paulo's personal tutor would most likely explore with Paulo ways of facilitating his return to his home country to be with his grandmother at the end of her life. Most courses allow students to interrupt their studies when they have major personal crises and restart them later, once the crisis has been resolved. While students are often reluctant to interrupt, in hindsight most feel it was the right decision. Sometimes, it is not possible for a student to interrupt, perhaps because of financial reasons or because the course regulations have a limit on time allowed to complete a course. If it is not possible for Paulo to interrupt his studies, his personal tutor would probably explore ways of supporting him while he remained at the university: this might even include referral to the counselling service. His personal tutor would probably also explore practical issues such as helping him obtain extensions on assignment deadlines or preparing a case for 'extenuating circumstances' in case he performed poorly in his assessments.

C

Laila's personal tutor will probably want to get to the root of the problem, as there are many reasons for students missing placements. Once the root of the problem has been established, her personal tutor can advise on a specific plan of action.

Sometimes, the root of the problem is students not understanding the professional obligations of nursing, such as good timekeeping and the importance of being courteous (eg by apologising if late), but, more often than not, it is down to personal issues such as disillusionment with the course or relationship problems. If it's about not understanding professional obligations, any feedback given to Laila is likely to be stern and straight to the point. It is important that Laila is in no doubt about the importance of professional standards in nursing. If it's about disillusionment, Laila's personal tutor might explain that most students get disillusioned at some point and they might further explore the situation to see if there are particular issues with this specific placement, such as poor supervision or intense workload. If it's about relationship problems, the student may well be signposted to other support services in the university, such as the counselling service.

D

Mark could raise this with a module lecturer or his personal tutor. They will most likely explain to Mark the NMC Code's professional requirement to raise concerns but will understand the predicament he finds himself in. They are likely to offer suggestions as to how he can fulfil his professional obligation to raise concerns while at the same time protecting himself from repercussions.

E

Shazia would benefit from discussing this with her personal tutor; it is a good case for a reflective discussion, not only in terms of how Shazia felt herself, but how she felt she was treated by the ward manager. The personal tutor would most likely explore ways in which Shazia might address such issues in the future while still maintaining a passion for nursing. Her personal tutor might also sensitively explore with Shazia whether she wanted to challenge – maybe even formally complain about – the ward manager's comments.

Getting the most from tutorials

Be prepared

The lecturer's time is undoubtedly very limited, so spend time thinking about how you can make the best use of this valuable one-to-one, face-to-face meeting time. It is a good idea to prepare by making some notes or forming some focused questions.

Ask the right questions

There are different types of question in English. See Chapter 1 for a detailed list and explanation of these. The type of question you use can have an impact on the interaction between you and the lecturer, and on how you are perceived. Understanding the difference between 'closed' and 'open' questions can be very helpful. These question types are discussed in detail in Chapter 1 of this book, but some examples relevant to tutorials are given below.

CROSS REFERENCE

Chapter 1, Professional speaking skills, Questioning techniques

- **'Closed'** or **'yes/no'** questions usually only require a one-word, or at least short, answer, eg:

  'Would it be better to start my essay with some background and contextual information?'

  'Is cognitive-behavioural therapy useful for people who self-harm?'

- **'Open'** or **'wh-'** questions usually elicit a more expansive answer, eg:

  'How should I start my essay?'

  'What interventions are useful for people who self-harm?'

Reflection

Both types of question outlined above have their place in any conversation, including the one you have with a lecturer in a tutorial. However, think about how the different types of question might affect the interaction in a tutorial and how they might affect the perceptions of the lecturer.

1)

'Would it be better to start my essay with some background and contextual information?'

versus

'How should I start my essay?'

2)

'Is cognitive-behavioural therapy useful for people who self-harm?'

versus

'What interventions are useful for people who self-harm?'

Discussion of reflection

In this case, the closed questions may have some advantages (though this does depend on the particular context):

- They are usually easier and quicker to deal with, and tutorial time is usually quite limited.

- They can show the lecturer that you have already done some thinking yourself. The open questions in this case put the onus on the lecturer and ask them to do your thinking for you. The closed questions show that you have done some thinking yourself, and are now merely making good use of the expertise of the lecturer. It indicates that you are taking responsibility for your own learning, and that you are trying to learn independently. This will probably reflect positively on you and help facilitate a better relationship with the lecturer.

Check understanding

It can be difficult to take everything in when you are in a tutorial, so try to check understanding at certain points. You can do this by asking questions:

'Do you mean…?'
'Is that the same as…?'
'What was the name of the book you mentioned?'
'Could you just explain what you mean by…?'
'Can I just ask you about that last point…?'

You can also try to briefly summarise what you think is the main message and ask for confirmation:

'If I understand correctly, the term psychosis includes…'
'Can I just check that I understand? Are you saying that…?'
'So, you're suggesting I compare these two approaches using the framework outlined in…?'

You can also state more directly that you haven't understood something by using the following polite phrases:

'I didn't quite catch what you said about…'
'I'm afraid I don't quite understand what you mean when you say that…'

Be assertive – but not rude!

Do not be afraid to be assertive. There might be points of disagreement between you and the tutor or lecturer, and this should be openly acknowledged. You just need to be careful that assertiveness doesn't tip over into rudeness. Negative questions can help 'soften' this type of exchange:

'Isn't it true that…?'
'Wouldn't it be better to…?'
'Don't you think that it would be better to…?'
'Doesn't that depend on…?'

And the use of 'pivot' phrases to disagree can also be effective:

'I see what you mean, but…'
'I understand what you're saying, I just thought that…'

Notice the use of 'softening' words such as 'just', 'quite' and 'really'. This is discussed in more detail in Chapter 4 of this book.

CROSS REFERENCE

Chapter 4, Participating in group seminars and meetings, Mind your language

Take notes

It is a good idea to take a few notes during a tutorial. Lecturers will be expecting you to do this. Later, you can review the notes to make sure you've understood everything. If there are action points to follow up on, or there's anything that doesn't seem to make sense, email as soon as possible ('Can I just confirm that…?') 'Could you please send the reference you mentioned…?') while the conversation is still fresh in both your minds.

Summary

This chapter has explained the different types of tutorial that can form part of your university studies. It has discussed the important role that individual tutorials play in your academic and personal development, particularly in terms of personalised direction and feedback. It has provided guidance to help you make the most of this valuable time with your lecturers at university, focusing on a number of useful interactional and linguistic strategies.

References

QAA (Quality Assurance Agency for Higher Education) (2011) Explaining Contact Hours: Guidance for Institutions Providing Public Information about Higher Education in the UK [online]. Available at: http://dera.ioe.ac.uk/10451/7/contact_hours_Redacted.pdf (accessed 12 September 2018).

Chapter 6
Networking

Learning outcomes

After reading this chapter, you will:

- have developed a better understanding of the concept of networking;

- have developed an understanding of the role that networking can play in your academic and professional life;

- have developed strategies to help you network effectively in both face-to-face and virtual contexts;

- be better equipped to manage the opportunities and challenges presented by social media and other online platforms.

This chapter explores the role of networking in your nursing studies. Networking involves interacting with other people in order to exchange information and knowledge, or to develop social and professional contacts and associations. This chapter will explore the different networking platforms – whether face to face or virtual – available to students and nurses. It will allow you to reflect on your current networking skills, and on your current relationship with social media and other online platforms. It will explore what kind of networking-related activities and behaviours are appropriate for students and nurses, with particular reference to the NMC Code (2015). It will also help you to refine your networking skills so that you can use them to good effect in your academic and professional life.

Opportunities and challenges related to networking

There are a number of opportunities and challenges associated with networking. Networking activities can:

- provide **mutual academic and professional support**;
- facilitate the **sharing of information and knowledge**;
- present **opportunities for collaboration**;
- support **personal and professional development**.

Challenges associated with networking activities relate to:

- the need for a certain degree of **confidence** and well-developed '**soft skills**', ie **communication skills** and **people skills**, also referred to as **interpersonal skills** (as opposed to technical or clinical skills);

- widely reported **concerns surrounding social media and other online platforms**, mainly related to **security** and **reputation**.

These opportunities and challenges will be discussed in later sections of this chapter.

Different types of networking

There are many different ways to network as a student and as a nurse. **Conferences** are a long-standing, well-established forum for academics, students and professionals to come together to share research, experience, knowledge and ideas. Such gatherings provide an obvious opportunity for people to network both formally and informally. Professional organisations, such as the Royal College of Nursing, also provide networking opportunities through local and national **meetings**, as well as conferences. Since the start of the 21st century, **social media** and other **online platforms** have also become increasingly important for networking.

Nursing students come to university with varying degrees of exposure to the different networking platforms, both for professional and for social purposes. The following task allows you to reflect on your current knowledge and experience of these platforms.

Task

1) Complete the table according to your experience of these types of networking, ie:

a) how often you do these things;
b) your purpose in using them;
c) your likes and dislikes.

	a) HOW OFTEN			b) PURPOSE		c) LIKES/ DISLIKES		
	OFTEN	SOME-TIMES	NEVER	PERSONAL USE	USE FOR STUDY OR WORK	😊	😐	🙁
Conferences								
Professional organisation meetings								
Traditional sports/social clubs or societies								

	a) HOW OFTEN			b) PURPOSE		c) LIKES/ DISLIKES		
	OFTEN	SOME-TIMES	NEVER	PERSONAL USE	USE FOR STUDY OR WORK	☺	😐	☹
Political/ activist groups								
Facebook								
LinkedIn								
Twitter								
Instagram								
YouTube								
Snapchat								
Whatsapp								
Chatrooms								
Discussion boards*								
Writing/ reading blogs**								
Nursing blogs or chatrooms								

* for example on a VLE such as Blackboard or Moodle
** online public diaries

2) Discuss and compare your table with other students. Discuss the reasons behind your usage and preferences.

3) Now you've heard about other people's experience and preferences, are there any forms of networking which you might think about doing, or doing more (or less!), or doing differently?

4) What factors do you consider when creating your **profile** for the social media sites that you use?

5) Look at the profile in the following case study. Do you think this is a good online profile for a student nurse? Give reasons.

Case study

Example online professional profile

Tom Kowalski

22 years old, student nurse (child field), University of Anytown

I am a compassionate second-year student nurse and proud father of two daughters. I'm a keen scuba diver and avid sci-fi reader. I am heavily involved in supporting and fundraising for my local Macmillan Centre.

I am particularly interested in paediatric oncology and am hoping to work in this area on qualifying. I have some basic web design and coding skills that have sparked an interest in the potential role of apps and other digital technology in supporting children with long-term conditions, as well as their families.

I'm looking to network with other children's nurses and/or those interested in paediatric oncology and/or digital health for children and families.

Email: tomk22@xyzmail.net

Nursing networking sites

Some particularly useful networking sites for nurses include:

- the **@WeNurses** Twitter group (and its subgroups such as @WeCYPnurses, @WeMHNurses, @WeLDnurses, @WeStudentNurse and @WeMidwives); see also the #WeCommunities website at www.wecommunities.org;
- other Twitter accounts that might be useful include those associated with the NHS (eg NHS England @NHSEngland, NHS Improvement @NHSImprovement, NHS Digital @NHSDigital, and individual NHS trusts), regulatory bodies (eg the NMC @nmcnews, the Care Quality Commission @CareQualityComm, the National Institute for Health and Care Excellence @NICEcomms), professional bodies (eg the School and Public Health Nurses' Association @SAPHNAteam, the RCN @theRCN, the Mental Health Nurses' Association @Unite_MHNA) and relevant government departments (eg Public Health England @PHE_uk, the Department of Health and Social Care @DHSCgovuk, the Scottish Government @scotgov, the Welsh Government @WelshGovernment, the Northern Ireland Assembly @niassembly);
- nursing and Midwifery forums at **The Student Room** website: www.thestudentroom.co.uk;
- specific subgroups within **Facebook** (your course, university or even specific field of nursing may have its own Facebook page);
- the specialist forums at the Royal College of Nursing: www.rcn.org.uk/get-involved/forums.

Networking and the NMC Code

All nurses and student nurses must make sure that their activities and behaviour are in line with the NMC Code (2015).

Reflection

Look at the extracts from the NMC Code (2015) below.

How do you think these broad principles could relate to the networking activities you discussed earlier in the chapter (face to face and virtual)?

1.1 Treat people with kindness, respect and compassion.

5.1 Respect a person's right to privacy in all aspects of their care.

7.5 Be able to communicate clearly and effectively in English.

8.2 Maintain effective communication with colleagues.

10.6 Collect, treat and store all data and research findings appropriately.

20.5 Use all forms of spoken, written and digital communication (including social media and networking sites) responsibly.

20.6 Stay objective and have clear professional boundaries at all times with people in your care (including those who have been in your care in the past), their families and carers.

21.3 Act with honesty and integrity in any financial dealings you have with everyone you have a professional relationship with, including people in your care.

These principles are discussed in more detail in the rest of the chapter, particularly in relation to social media.

Conferences

Conferences are forums where academics, students and professionals gather to share research, experience, knowledge and ideas. There are usually a series of presentations where people present their research findings or describe some aspect of their work. There will usually be a **plenary** (a session attended by all participants of the conference) at the beginning and the end of the conference, usually led by a distinguished academic or professional in the field. People will then usually split into smaller groups for the other sessions. Formal academic **presentations** will often run alongside more informal **workshops** and **meetings**.

All of these provide opportunities to meet and talk to people with similar academic and professional interests and concerns. For example, presentations usually end by opening up the floor with a question-and-answer session, and workshops provide important opportunities for group discussion. But it is often outside of these scheduled events that some of the most important networking occurs. Coffee and lunch breaks (and sometimes formal dinners or even excursions at longer conferences) are an excellent opportunity for people to catch up with acquaintances or former colleagues. They are also a chance to meet new people. Conferences are thus important networking platforms in addition to being important for the advancement of knowledge and the enhancement of professional practice.

The first conference you attend might feel a bit intimidating or even 'cliquey', but really what you're seeing is the effect of networking: these people who seem to know each other so well may also have been intimidated at their first conference, but they were brave enough to start a conversation that led to a professional relationship or even a personal friendship. There are a number of ways to be proactive: you might decide to speak to one of the presenters, or someone whose post-presentation question intrigued you; you might talk to someone from a particular institution or organisation (information often included on name tags), perhaps in relation to professional development.

Professional organisations

Many nursing and health-related professional organisations provide opportunities for networking, whether face to face or online. Examples include organisations such as the Royal College of Nursing (who have a big members' gathering every year called 'Congress'), the School and Public Health Nurses' Association, the Mental Health Nurses Association (hosted by the trade union, Unite), the Royal College of Midwives, the British Psychological Society, and the British Association of Critical Care Nurses. You will probably need to pay a fee, ie a 'subscription' to become a member of these organisations, but many offer cheaper rates for students.

The internet and social media

Most of you will probably have already developed a range of habits and skills related to internet and social media use. These may include:

- communicating through social networking sites (eg Facebook, LinkedIn, Twitter);
- sharing online content, eg text, photos, video and audio files (eg on Twitter, Instagram, YouTube, WhatsApp, Snapchat);
- creating or using websites;
- writing or following blogs;
- contributing to discussion boards (eg on VLEs).

It is likely that you will be able to draw on this experience to develop your professional networking skills. However, you may also have to reflect on your internet and social media use, and possibly adapt your activity and behaviour to suit your new academic and professional context. You are no doubt aware of the current spate of debates surrounding the internet and social media. In fact, there have been a number of recent media reports on nurses who have been disciplined for inappropriate behaviour on social media, including lapses in professionalism and breaches of confidentiality. For example, a mental health nurse was removed from the NMC Register in 2016 for offensive Facebook posts (BBC, 2016).

The following quote from an editorial in the *Journal of Clinical Nursing* (Jones and Hayter, 2013, p 1495) serves to remind how times change, and how nurses need to adapt to those changes:

> 'As students several decades ago we recall being told 'don't talk about patients or colleagues in the hospital lift – you never know who is listening.'

At the time evoked by the authors, the lift scenario was one of the few in which a nurse could put themselves at risk of being overheard talking inappropriately. Today, with the proliferation of social media platforms, any inappropriate talk could reach large numbers of people scattered far and wide, rather than just those people standing over your shoulder in the lift.

Social media and the NMC Code

The big advantage of social media for nurses is that it offers the opportunity to 'connect with colleagues the world over in a professional dialogue' (Jones and Hayter, 2013, p 1495). A good example of this is the way in which a nurse in Bolton can access a live feed of a conference in Chicago on Twitter as it happens, perhaps viewing PowerPoint slides or reading about audience reactions.

The NMC lists the benefits of social media for nurses, midwives and students as follows (nd, p 4):

- building and maintaining professional relationships;
- establishing or accessing nursing and midwifery support networks and being able to discuss specific issues, interests, research and clinical experience with other healthcare professionals globally;
- being able to access resources for continuing professional development (CPD).

However, the NMC is also at pains to point out that social media can only be a successful networking tool if it is used responsibly.

Using social media and the internet responsibly

Social media and the internet are useful, powerful tools which can inform us, entertain us and connect us. But they can also easily get out of control and lead to misunderstanding, embarrassment and even danger. This can cause problems in any aspect of your life. However, as a student and as a professional, the stakes are potentially very high. Irresponsible use of social media, including unlawful or unprofessional behaviour, can put your registration at risk. Behaviour of this type can include (NMC, nd, p 3):

- sharing confidential information inappropriately;
- posting pictures of patients or service users without their consent;
- posting inappropriate comments about patients or service users;
- bullying, intimidating or exploiting people;
- encouraging violence or self-harm;
- inciting hatred or discrimination;
- pursuing relationships with patients or service users;
- stealing personal information or using someone else's identity.

Task

Make notes on how the actions and behaviours above contravene the NMC Code principles discussed at the beginning of this chapter. They may contravene more than one principle. One example has been added.

NMC CODE	ACTION/ BEHAVIOUR CONTRAVENING CODE	NOTES
1.1 Treat people with kindness, respect and compassion	Sharing confidential information inappropriately	We especially need to help patients 'uphold their dignity' (NMC, 2015, p 4)
5.1 Respect a person's right to privacy in all aspects of their care	Sharing confidential information inappropriately	We are all sensitive about aspects of our health and private life and would not wish everyone to know about these. 'As a nurse or midwife, you owe a duty of confidentiality to all those who are receiving care.' (NMC, 2015, p 6)
7.5 Be able to communicate clearly and effectively in English		
8.2 Maintain effective communication with colleagues		

NMC CODE	ACTION/ BEHAVIOUR CONTRAVENING CODE	NOTES
10.6 Collect, treat and store all data and research findings appropriately	Sharing confidential information inappropriately	And so 'respect people's right to privacy and confidentiality' (NMC, 2015, p 6). These rights are upheld by law – see new GDPR regulations (2018)
20.5 Use all forms of spoken, written and digital communication (including social media and networking sites) responsibly		
20.6 Stay objective and have clear professional boundaries at all times with people in your care (including those who have been in your care in the past), their families and carers		
21.3 Act with honesty and integrity in any financial dealings you have with everyone you have a professional relationship with, including people in your care		

When using social media and the internet in general, it is important to be aware at all times of your 'presence, footprints or image' (Jones and Hayter, 2013, p 1495), ie how you will appear to colleagues, patients, or prospective employers. It is also important to understand that patients are also users of social media, and they may in fact attempt to contact you though social media. The perceived informality of this medium can make it difficult to maintain professional boundaries. In fact, professional networking on social media does not normally include adding patients you have worked with to your social media accounts, even if they request it (see NMC Code, 2015, 20.6).

First and foremost, it is essential that your use of social media adheres to the regulations and guidelines issued by universities and employers, as well as by professional bodies, in particular the NMC. There are also general 'rules' of behaviour which can help you use social media and the internet in a responsible way.

Netiquette

It is not possible to cover every instance of social media use that you will encounter, but there are 'rules of thumb' that you can follow to help you to navigate this complex world safely, professionally and effectively. These rules are sometimes referred to as **'netiquette'** (a portmanteau of 'internet' and 'etiquette' – good manners in social interaction). The rules of netiquette can help to promote the professional behaviour expected of students and those working in the care professions such as nursing. They can help protect you and others from harm and embarrassment. The following **top tips** box lists some netiquette rules which can guide you towards posting responsibly on social media.

Top tips

Posting responsibly

- **Be social media savvy.** Be aware of how the medium you are posting on works, and how to control any filters or privacy settings. Be clear about what other people will see or hear when you post. Take any action you can to protect yourself and others.

- **Think before you post.** You may come to regret an unguarded comment or an embarrassing photo. These could be seen by a prospective employer, for example. Also, avoid using social media to let off steam or complain about work or colleagues.

- **Post with integrity.** Post when you are in the right frame of mind and with the right intentions. Don't post after a night out, or when you are upset, for example. Also, avoid plagiarism, just as you would in an academic essay or presentation. Credit photos and cite authors. Don't pass off anything as your own if it isn't.

- **Post appropriately.** The use of social media spans our professional and personal lives, and this can sometimes lead us to blur the boundaries between them. While nurses can find social media a valuable forum for discussion of some of the frustrations and challenges of the workplace, it is also important to understand where the acceptable limits of such conversations lie (Jones and Hayter, 2013). Your default tone should be one of politeness and restraint – though of course, there are times when it is fine to be excited or effusive – when you are congratulating someone on an achievement, for example. Also remember the NMC requirement to 'communicate clearly' (2015, p 7). This means paying attention to grammar and punctuation. You should also avoid 'text language' when posting professionally or on a platform that is publicly accessible.

- **Post professionally.** If in doubt, consider the **NMC Code**, in particular, the requirement to **'uphold the reputation of your profession at all times'** (2015, p 15) and **'uphold your position as a registered nurse of midwife'** (2015, p 16). Ask yourself if your post lives up to these standards of conduct. And remember that some private platforms may be more public than you think. Many of us working with students are aware of cases in which students have posted offensive things about lecturers on a closed Facebook group only for other members of that group to take offence, print a hard copy of the posting for evidence, and then report the student to the university. Also, be aware that deleting a post does not necessarily mean it has not left a footprint.

Summary

This chapter has outlined the concept of networking and explored some of the different networking platforms available to students and nurses. It has looked at some of the behaviours and activities associated with networking, both face to face and online, and discussed what is considered to be appropriate for students and nurses, with particular reference to the NMC Code (2015). It has suggested ways in which you, as a student nurse, can refine your networking skills so that you can use them to good effect in your academic and professional life, as well as your personal life.

References

BBC (2016) Clacton Mental Health Nurse Struck Off for Facebook Posts, 26 November [online]. Available at: www.bbc.co.uk/news/uk-england-essex-38102949 (accessed 15 September 2018).

Jones, C and Hayter, M (2013) Editorial: Social Media Use by Nurses and Midwives: A 'Recipe for Disaster' or a 'Force for Good'? *Journal of Clinical Nursing*, 22: 1495–6.

NMC (Nursing and Midwifery Council) (2015) *The Code: Professional Standards of Practice and Behaviour for Nurses and Midwives* [online]. Available at: www.nmc. org.uk/globalassets/sitedocuments/standards/nmc-standards-for-competence-for-registered-nurses.pdf (accessed 18 July 2018).

NMC (Nursing and Midwifery Council) (nd) *Guidance on Using Social Media Responsibly* [online]. Available at: www.nmc.org.uk/globalassets/sitedocuments/nmc-publications/social-media-guidance.pdf (accessed 13 September 2018).

Appendix 1
Academic levels at university

UNDERGRADUATE STUDY			
England, Wales, Northern Ireland	Scotland	Award	Notes
Level 4	Level 7	Certificate of Higher Education (CertHE)	
Level 5	Level 8	Diploma of Higher Education (DipHE) Foundation Degree (FdD)	Up until 2010, minimum academic qualification for nurses
Level 6	Level 9	Ordinary Bachelor Degree eg BSc Nursing	Minimum academic qualification for nurses and midwives; common exit point in Scotland
	Level 10	Bachelor Degree with Honours eg BSc (Hons) in Nursing Studies, BNurs (Hons), BMidwif (Hons)	Usual academic qualification for nurses and midwives in England, Wales and Northern Ireland
POSTGRADUATE STUDY			
Level 7	Level 11	Masters Degree, eg MSc, MA, MPhil Postgraduate Certificate or Diploma (PGCert; PGDip)	Minimum academic qualification for Advanced Practitioners
Level 8	Level 12	Research Doctorate (PhD) Professional Doctorate eg DNurs, MD, ClinPsychD	Recommended qualification for Advanced Practitioners who are Nurse Consultants

Appendix 2
Key phrases in assignments

analyse	Mostly levels 5 and 6, especially with the word 'critically'; rarely level 4	Look at the concepts and ideas under discussion in depth; the addition of 'critically' means look at the concepts and ideas in depth **and** with a critical eye
assess	All levels, though common at lower levels	Make comments about the value/importance of the concepts and ideas under discussion
compare	All levels, though common at lower levels	Look for similarities between the concepts and ideas under discussion
contrast	All levels, though common at lower levels	Look for differences between the concepts and ideas under discussion; often used with 'compare' (see above)
define	All levels, though common at lower levels	State precisely what is meant by a particular issue, theory or concept
discuss	Level 5 and above; sometimes level 4	Give reasons for and against; investigate and examine by argument
evaluate	Mostly levels 5 and 6, especially with the word 'critically'	Weigh up the arguments surrounding an issue, using your own opinions and, more importantly, reference to the work of others
illustrate	All levels	Make clear by the use of examples
outline	All levels, though tends to be used with the lower levels	Give the main features of
review	All levels, though 'critically review' would imply level 5 and above	Extract relevant information from a document or set of documents
state	All levels, though tends to be used with the lower levels	Present in a clear, concise form
summarise	All levels, though tends to be used with the lower levels	Give an account of all the main points of the concepts and ideas under discussion
with reference to	All levels	Use a specific context, issue or concept to make the meaning clear

Appendix 3
English language references

This is not meant to be an exhaustive list of resources, but rather a selection of those that we have found most useful in our work with students.

Dictionaries

There are many online dictionaries, but if you prefer to feel the weight of one in your hands, then Chambers is a good choice:

Chambers 21st Century Dictionary (1999) Edinburgh: Chambers Harrap Publishers Ltd.

A good online dictionary, especially for students whose first language is not English, is the Cambridge Dictionary. The definitions are very clear and easy to understand, and there is an excellent pronunciation tool for students whose first language is not English:

Cambridge Dictionary [online]. Available at: http://dictionary.cambridge.org (accessed 19 October 2018).

Grammar books

Caplan, N (2012) *Grammar Choices for Graduate and Professional Writers*. Ann Arbor, MI: University of Michigan Press.

Caplan's book is aimed at postgraduate students (known as 'graduate' students in the USA, where this book is published). Nevertheless, if you are looking for a systematic analysis of English grammar in the context of academic English, you may find this book very useful. It contains many clear examples of grammar in use in real-life academic writing.

Hewings, M (2015) *Advanced Grammar in Use*. 3rd ed. Cambridge: Cambridge University Press.

Murphy, R (2015) *English Grammar in Use*. 4th ed. Cambridge: Cambridge University Press.

Murphy, R (2015) *Essential Grammar in Use*. 4th ed. Cambridge: Cambridge University Press.

The Grammar in Use series is particularly useful for students whose first language is not English. The books present each grammar point in a clear and systematic way, and provide exercises and a self-study answer key. There are also lots of multimedia features in recent editions.

Other resources

Academic Phrasebank [online]. Available at: www.phrasebank.manchester.ac.uk (accessed 19 October 2018).

Academic Word List [online]. Available at: www.victoria.ac.nz/lals/resources/ academicwordlist (accessed 19 October 2018).

Baily, S (2011) *Academic Writing for International Students of English*. 3rd ed. Oxon: Routledge.

Bottomley, J (2014) *Academic Writing for International Students of Science*. Oxon: Routledge.

Peck, J and Cole, M (2012) *Write it Right: The Secrets of Effective Writing*. 2nd ed. New York: Palgrave Macmillan.

Swales, J and Feak, C (2012) *Academic Writing for Graduate Students: Essential Tasks and Skills*. 3rd ed. Michigan: Michigan ELT.

Answer key

Chapter 1, Professional speaking skills

Being a good communicator

Task: Active listening (page 12)

1) Acknowledging what the patient has said; restating and reflecting back to the patient what they have told you to check that you understand correctly.

2) First part of the response demonstrates active listening – echoing, clarification; second part explores the issue in an attempt to be empathic.

3) Example of active listening by both the patient and the nurse, which is typical in flowing conversations; involves restating and clarifying.

4) Active listening allows nurse to pick up on patient's desire to eat more healthily; acknowledges the patient wants to change and starts exploring this issue further.

Chapter 2, Professional writing skills

Record keeping

Task: Use and misuse of abbreviations and acronyms (page 27)

> Mrs Sutton was admitted to Ward 37 by Staff Nurse [saves confusion with other roles with the same initials, eg Student Nurse, Senior Nurse] Rosenbaum at 13:00 hours [24 hour clock format prevents confusion]. She reported that she had been passing faeces that looked 'black, like tar' and had had a couple of episodes of vomiting that looked like ground coffee. She has experienced stomach problems on and off in the past for which she took 75mg of over-the-counter [written in full rather than 'otc'] ranitidine [Zantac is the trade name for ranitidine] as needed [prn, short for pro re nata, is a Latin term meaning 'as required']. Blood sample taken for full blood count [this is what 'FBC' means]. Awaiting urgent endoscopy [used instead of 'GI scope' which is short for gastro-intestinal scope].

Writing reports

Task (pages 30–31)

1) Background – B

What are the issues? – A

What needs to happen? – C

2) A. a) shape; b) diverse

B. a) kept pace with; b) approximately; c) rates; d) estimated; e) although;
   f) agency nurses

C. a) retention; b) ensure; c) vital

Writing reports
Task (page 32)

A key objective of any future immigration system should be ensuring that the UK can attract and retain the highly skilled nursing workforce required to provide quality care which meets patient need. Internationally recruited nurses have made an important contribution to this goal while enhancing the cultural diversity of the profession and facilitating a rich exchange of skills and experience.

Writing official letters
Task (page 33)

1) Which address is that of a) the sender and b) the recipient?

The sender's is in the top left-hand corner; the recipient's is on the right, slightly lower down the page.

2) What does 're' (first line of the letter) mean?

'Regarding'. This is a common way of starting an official letter as it makes the topic immediately clear; in this case, the patient's name is given prominence.

3) The letter starts with 'Dear Dr Other' and ends with 'Yours sincerely'. When would you end a letter with 'Yours faithfully'?

See the **Top tips** box immediately following the letter.

4) What is the purpose of the letter?

The purpose is to inform the doctor who has referred the patient to the community mental health team about the patient's state of mind and the treatment that has been recommended.

5) Who will read the letter?

The doctor who made the referral and Mr Person – we can see that, although the letter is addressed to Dr Other, Mr Person is copied in (cc) at the end of the letter, which means he will receive an exact copy (cc is short for 'carbon copy') of the letter.

6) Is the language used in the letter suitable for all readers?

The language is formal but accessible. The letter has a conversational, narrative style which makes it easy to relate to and follow (most of us are used to story-telling in books and on TV). Mr Person, as well as the doctor, will be able to understand easily.

7) Does the letter follow the Academy of Royal Medical Colleges guidelines (2018) discussed earlier?

As Mr Person will read the letter, the Academy guidelines are relevant. The letter mostly avoids medical jargon and uses 'plain English'. There are no Latin terms and most of the words used are part of most people's vocabulary. The words 'ruminate' and 'ideation' are not everyday words, but they are used with explanation and exemplification. There are no acronyms – the term 'cognitive-behavioural programme', rather than 'CBT', is used. The letter is scrupulously transparent – events are clearly specified, statements are carefully attributed (with some speech marks indicating the exact words used). The tone is sensitive to Mr and Mrs Person's challenging situation, and tries to convey their feelings rather than putting words in their mouth. There is no stigmatising of Mr Person's condition. He is taken seriously and spoken about in an objective, respectful manner.

Chapter 3, Academic presentations and public speaking

Giving effective academic presentations, Research and preparation

Task: Organising information and ideas (page 44)

All should start with an introduction:

- Introduction
  - about myself;
  - aims/structure of the session;
  - any ground rules (eg ask questions at end or it's fine to interrupt).

They should end with:

- wrap up/summary and any questions;
- a 'take-home message' if possible.

Possible structures:

1) **The nursing family in the current NHS**
   - The nursing family

- Explore workers loosely categorised as 'nurses':
  - Healthcare assistants
  - Nursing associates
  - Registered nurses
  - Advanced Practice Nurses
- Outline debate over what a nurse is, focusing on the registered nurse (RN) and claims of attempts to 'dumb down' nursing
- Argument that RNs have to be graduates

- Workforce and skill mix
  - Necessity of skill mix
  - Skill mix and patient safety: safe staffing
- The future nurse
  - New NMC standard
  - What the NHS might look like in the future and what it will require of the nursing family

2) **The role of nurses in palliative care**
- What is palliative care?
  - Definitions
  - Facts and figures
  - Provision of services
- The role of nurses in palliative care
  - Acute vs. community nursing
  - Sub-specialties, eg cancer care, children's palliative care, palliative care in dementia
  - Skills required of palliative care nurses
- Examples of nurses as leaders in palliative care, eg Macmillan nurses

3) **Anxiety in children and young people**
- What is anxiety and why it is an issue in children and young people (C&YP)?
  - Definitions
  - Prevalence/public health aspects
  - Impact on C&YP, eg school, peer-relationships
- How to help C&YP with anxiety
  - Medical treatments, eg medication
  - Psychological treatments, eg cognitive-behaviour therapy
  - Self-management approaches
- The nurse's role in helping C&YP with anxiety

Chapter 4, Participating in group seminars and meetings

The role of seminars in universities

Task (pages 60–61)

4)

a) Seminars provide an opportunity to follow up on a lecture. They allow you to demonstrate your understanding of the topic, and to clarify anything that you didn't understand from the lecture itself. **both**

b) Seminar discussion can enable you to forge a deeper understanding of ideas and concepts. **thinking**

c) Seminar discussions can be good preparation for essays, exams and other assessments, as they provide a space for you to test your understanding and ideas, and work out how to express them in a clear, convincing way. **both**

d) Seminars provide an opportunity to learn from people with different knowledge, background, experience and perspectives from your own. **thinking**

e) Seminar discussion may lead you to change, develop or adapt your opinions and ideas as you come into contact with others' views. **thinking**

f) Some seminar activities can help you develop your problem-solving skills. **thinking**

g) Frequent participation in seminars can help you become more confident about public speaking. **communication**

h) Seminars can help you become more confident about discussing complex issues and ideas. **communication**

i) Seminars can help you improve the way you interact with others in a group setting. **communication**

j) Seminar skills are transferable skills which can help you in your professional practice, for example in teamwork and meetings with colleagues. **communication**

The conventions of seminars

Task (page 64)

1) 'Wouldn't you say that poverty is a factor here?' **politely/cautiously challenging/contributing**

2) 'Yes, but what about parity of esteem between mental and physical health?' **politely challenging/contributing**

3) 'But surely that's the role of government?' **politely challenging/disagreeing**

4) 'What do you think Claire?' **inviting participation**

5) 'As Mia said, the policy seems to disadvantage family carers and advantage the government, who essentially get care from relatives free of charge.' **acknowledging contributions/reformulating**

6) 'I think Portugal is a good example of somewhere where drug addiction is seen as a health issue rather than a criminal issue.' **making a contribution to the discussion**

7) 'Did you say you worked with people with dementia on your placement, Lia?' **inviting participation**

8) 'Could I just add something to what Dan said?' **acknowledging contributions and building on them**

9) 'Aren't we forgetting the impact of peer pressure?' **politely challenging/ contributing**

10) 'But isn't that more an issue of compliance? Or is it "concordance" or "adherence" that we use now?' **politely challenging/contributing/clarifying/ checking**

11) 'I take your point, but what about patient autonomy?' **politely disagreeing**

12) 'I see what you mean, but why is that important?' **politely challenging/ disagreeing**

13) 'According to one of the studies we were asked to look at, there is some evidence to suggest that the treatment can be effective if it is combined with other therapies.' **supporting ideas with evidence**

14) 'But didn't that study have a really small sample size?' **challenging**

15) 'I didn't quite catch what you said about the stats.' **asking for clarification**

16) 'Sorry, could you just explain what you mean by "alternative therapies"? I ask because lots of different therapies with widely varying evidence bases get lumped together under that heading.' **asking for clarification**

17) 'I'm afraid I don't quite follow your point.' **asking for clarification**

18) 'So what you're saying is that we need to provide different types of support.' **reformulating/checking**

19) 'Yes, that's a really good example.' **acknowledging contributions**

20) 'Yes, I hadn't thought of that.' **acknowledging contributions**

21) 'Are you sure about that? It's not how I interpreted it.' **politely/cautiously disagreeing**

22) 'I don't really think that what you're suggesting is realistic, given the current financial crisis in the NHS.' **politely disagreeing**

23) 'Are we all agreed on that?' **reaching consensus**

Mind your language

Task (page 71)

2)

    A (ii)

    B (iii)

    C (i)

Index

Note: **bold** page numbers refer to tables.